Health Care Reform and Gastroenterology

Guest Editors

JOHN I. ALLEN, MD, MBA
MARK H. DELEGGE, MD

GASTROINTESTINAL ENDOSCOPY CLINICS OF NORTH AMERICA

www.giendo.theclinics.com

Consulting Editor
CHARLES J. LIGHTDALE, MD

January 2012 • Volume 22 • Number 1

SAUNDERS an imprint of ELSEVIER, Inc.

W.B. SAUNDERS COMPANY
A Division of Elsevier Inc.

1600 John F. Kennedy Blvd. ● Suite 1800 ● Philadelphia, Pennsylvania 19103-2899

http://www.giendo.theclinics.com

GASTROINTESTINAL ENDOSCOPY CLINICS OF NORTH AMERICA Volume 22, Number 1
January 2012 ISSN 1052-5157, ISBN-13: 978-1-4557-3865-6

Editor: Kerry Holland
Developmental Editor: Donald Mumford

Gastrointestinal Endoscopy Clinics of North America (ISSN 1052-5157) is published quarterly by Elsevier Inc., 360 Park Avenue South, New York, NY 10010-1710. Months of issue are January, April, July, and October. Business and Editorial Offices: 1600 John F. Kennedy Blvd., Suite 1800, Philadelphia, PA, 19103-2899. Periodicals postage paid at New York, NY and additional mailing offices. Subscription prices are $315.00 per year for US individuals, $441.00 per year for US institutions, $168.00 per year for US students and residents, $351.00 per year for Canadian individuals, $538.00 per year for Canadian institutions, $445.00 per year for international individuals, $538.00 per year for international institutions, and $234.00 per year for Canadian and foreign students/residents. To receive student/resident rate, orders must be accompanied by name of affiliated institution, date of term, and the *signature* of program/residency coordinator on institution letterhead. Orders will be billed at individual rate until proof of status is received. Foreign air speed delivery is included in all *Clinics* subscription prices. All prices are subject to change without notice. **POSTMASTER:** Send address change to *Gastrointestinal Endoscopy Clinics of North America*, Elsevier Health Sciences Division, Subscription Customer Service, 3251 Riverport Lane, Maryland Heights, MO 63043. **Customer Service: 1-800-654-2452 (US). From outside the United States, call 1-314-447-8871. Fax: 1-314-447-8029. E-mail: JournalsCustomerService-usa@elsevier.com (for print support) or JournalsOnlineSupport-usa@elsevier.com (for online support).**

Reprints. For copies of 100 or more, of articles in this publication, please contact the Commercial Reprints Department, Elsevier Inc., 360 Park Avenue South, New York, NY 10010-1710. Tel. (212) 633-3812; Fax: (212) 482-1935; E-mail: reprints@elsevier.com.

Gastrointestinal Endoscopy Clinics of North America is covered in *Excerpta Medica, MEDLINE/PubMed (Index Medicus), and MEDLINE/MEDLARS.*

Printed and bound by CPI Group (UK) Ltd, Croydon, CR0 4YY

Transferred to Digital Print 2012

Contributors

CONSULTING EDITOR

CHARLES J. LIGHTDALE, MD
Professor, Department of Medicine, Columbia University Medical Center, New York, New York

GUEST EDITORS

JOHN I. ALLEN, MD, MBA
Adjunct Professor of Medicine, University of Minnesota School of Medicine, Minnesota Gastroenterology PA, Minneapolis, Minnesota

MARK H. DELEGGE, MD
Professor of Medicine, Digestive Disease Center, Medical University of South Carolina, DeLegge Medical, Charleston, South Carolina

AUTHORS

JOHN I. ALLEN, MD, MBA
Adjunct Professor of Medicine, University of Minnesota School of Medicine, Minnesota Gastroenterology PA, Minneapolis, Minnesota

JOEL V. BRILL, MD
Predictive Health, LLC, Phoenix, Arizona

ROSS MCVICKER CLINCHY, PhD
Associate Dean for Administration, SUNY Downstate Medical Center, Dean's Office, School of Medicine, Brooklyn, New York

MARK H. DELEGGE, MD
Professor of Medicine, Digestive Disease Center, Medical University of South Carolina, and DeLegge Medical, Charleston, South Carolina

SPENCER D. DORN, MD, MPH
Assistant Professor of Medicine, Division of Gastroenterology and Hepatology, University of North Carolina School of Medicine, Chapel Hill, North Carolina

ROBERT A. GANZ, MD, FASGE
Minnesota Gastroenterology, PA, Bloomington; University of Minnesota, Minneapolis, Minnesota

RAJEEV JAIN, MD, FACP, AGAF
Texas Digestive Disease Consultants, Dallas, Texas

MICHAEL KOMAR, MD
Director, Geisinger Health System, and Gastroenterology Service Line Director, Danville, Pennsylvania

LAWRENCE R. KOSINSKI, MD, MBA, AGAF, FACG
Managing Partner, Illinois Gastroenterology Group, Elgin, Illinois

KLAUS MERGENER, MD, PhD, MBA
Partner, Digestive Health Specialists, Clinical Medical Director, Gastroenterology, MultiCare Health System, Tacoma, Washington

RAHUL S. NAYAK, MD, MBA
Physician Director of Patient Safety, Gastroenterology, Southwood; The Southeast Permanente Medical Group, Kaiser Permanente, Jonesboro, Georgia

EILEEN PATTEN, BA
Geisinger Health System, Danville, Pennsylvania

KIMBERLY M. PERSLEY, MD
Texas Digestive Disease Consultants, Dallas, Texas

ROBERT SMITH, MD
Medical Director, Adult Liver Transplant Program, Geisinger Health System, Danville, Pennsylvania

IAN L. TAYLOR, MD, PhD, AGAF
Senior Vice President for Biomedical Education and Research, and Dean of the College of Medicine, SUNY Downstate Medical Center, School of Medicine, Brooklyn, New York

SAMUEL R. WALTERS, BS
Director of Quality Measurement and Informatics, American Gastroenterological Association, Bethesda, Maryland

Contents

THE CLINICS ARE NOW AVAILABLE ONLINE!
Access your subscription at:
www.theclinics.com

Foreword

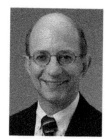

Charles J. Lightdale, MD
Consulting Editor

As a participant in the American Gastroenterological Association's Clinical Congress about a year ago, I had the opportunity to carefully review the program and attend many of the presentations. It was overall a splendid educational event aimed at practicing gastroenterologists, but what struck me as the most unique aspects of the Congress were the Practice Management Course and the Practice Skills Workshop. Here were assembled many of the senior thought leaders in gastroenterology providing practical advice to clinicians faced with bewildering choices on how to manage in changing times. I thought this might be the basis for a *Gastrointestinal Endoscopy Clinics of North America* issue, and I contacted the Course and Workshop Directors, Dr John Allen and Dr Mark DeLegge, to see if they might agree. Dr Allen responded with an even better proposal, more focused and compelling, "Health Care Reform and Gastroenterology 2012."

No matter what happens in politics or in the courts, it seems certain that the current systems of health care in the United States will evolve under pressure for cost reduction and the need to provide quality care to all citizens. It is difficult for gastroenterologists to understand how what they do will fit into the new systems and how they will have to adjust and adapt to be successful. This issue of the *Clinics* is critically relevant to these concerns at all levels, fellows-in-training, private practitioners, full-time hospital or clinic employees, and academics carrying out clinical research. This is truly a landmark issue with masterpiece articles that should be read and reread by clinical gastroenterologists and gastrointestinal endoscopists as we move forward into the challenging yet exciting new era.

Charles J. Lightdale, MD
Department of Medicine
Columbia University Medical Center
161 Fort Washington Avenue, Room 812
New York, NY 10032, USA

E-mail address:
CJL18@columbia.edu

Gastrointest Endoscopy Clin N Am 22 (2012) ix
doi:10.1016/j.giec.2011.09.003
1052-5157/12/$ – see front matter © 2012 Elsevier Inc. All rights reserved.

Preface

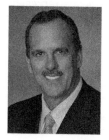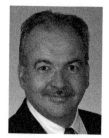

John I. Allen, MD, MBA   Mark H. DeLegge, MD
Guest Editors

The practice of Gastroenterology and the practice of United States medicine both are undergoing tectonic changes as a result of increasing economic constraints, patient demographics, the aging of practitioners, and, of course, the Patient Protection and Accountable Care Act (PPACA). Last January, at the American Gastroenterological Association Clinical Congress, Dr Charles Lightdale asked us to publish content from the Practice Management and Practice Skills Workshops. The Practice Management portion of the Congress is a 2-day course designed to update physicians and administrators on current changes in the practice of gastroenterology. The Practice Skills workshop is a course focused on GI Fellows transitioning into practice.

After we discussed the goals and objectives of the Practice Management course, it appeared obvious to all of us that a monograph outlining overarching changes and challenges facing gastroenterologists would be an excellent way to initiate the 2012 editions of *Gastrointestinal Endoscopy Clinics of North America*. We then set out to find the best authorities in gastroenterology and asked them to write about their special area of expertise. This monograph is a collection of articles focused on the major issues facing gastroenterologists as a result of PPACA.

PPACA, its related legislation, and the regulations emanating from these Congressional Acts will be game changers for all of us. The political climate during health care reform went from partisan to bitter partisan and the original area of agreement (expanding coverage to uninsured Americans) was lost in the 2,000-page bill finally passed by an arcane rule called "Reconciliation." PPACA was passed strictly along party lines. Never before has a bill of such far-reaching impact been passed without at least some bipartisan support. As parts of the bill trickle from legislation through regulation and into daily practice, there remain concerted legislative and judicial efforts to eradicate the bill either by piecemeal repeal or by complete elimination.

No matter what we believe individually about this bill or changes in medicine, we will all have to struggle with the chaotic picture that has become our reality. In the next decade we will see continued disappearance of our medical practices as we know

Gastrointest Endoscopy Clin N Am 22 (2012) xi–xii
doi:10.1016/j.giec.2011.09.005
1052-5157/12/$ – see front matter © 2012 Elsevier Inc. All rights reserved.

them and we will see large, integrated health care systems emerge. Whether independent GI practices of any size can continue to exist is an open question.

This edition of *Gastrointestinal Endoscopy Clinics of North America* represents a unique collection of expert opinions and descriptions focused on health care issues that impact gastroenterologists. We hope you find this monograph useful in framing your thoughts about how best to deliver patient-centered, high-quality, and, now, accountable care to your patients.

John I. Allen, MD, MBA
Minnesota Gastroenterology PA
5705 West Old Shakopee Road, Suite #150
Bloomington, MN 55437, USA

University of Minnesota School of Medicine
420 Delaware St, SE
Minneapolis, MN 55455, USA

Mark H. DeLegge, MD
Digestive Disease Center
Medical University of South Carolina
DeLegge Medical, 25 Courtenay Street, Suite 7100A
Charleston, SC 29425, USA

E-mail addresses:
jallen@mngastro.com (J.I. Allen)
deleggem@musc.edu (M.H. DeLegge)

Health Care Reform: 2012 Update

Spencer D. Dorn, MD, MPH

KEYWORDS

• Health care reform • Policy • Quality • Reimbursement

The deficiencies of the American health care system are well known. The recent White House Debt Commission opined that "federal health care spending represents our single largest fiscal challenge over the long-run."[1] Yet despite such massive spending, access to health care is limited,[2] quality of health care is uneven,[3] and health outcomes are often below par.[4] These problems are not new. By the early 1970s, after experts had declared a health care crisis, President Nixon emphasized that "The time for action is now."[5] Nonetheless, over the ensuing decades a combination of inaction and incrementalism limited major progress toward fixing health care.[6,7]

When President Barack Obama entered office it was by no means an auspicious moment to attempt sweeping policy changes. His administration faced soaring federal budget deficits, a unified front of opposition, and staunch resistance from special interest groups interested in preserving the status quo. In addition, opponent-led chants of "rationing," "death panels," and "government takeover," often drowned out efforts to explain how ordinary Americans would benefit from health care reform. Nonetheless, the Obama administration managed to successfully navigate around these obstacles and moved quickly to keep health care reform a top priority from the start. Within several months of entering office, the American Recovery and Reinvestment Act was passed and then signed; it committed $150 billion in health care investments, primarily in health information technology (HIT) and comparative effectiveness research (CER).[8] Over the following year the President assiduously campaigned for health care reform and left key policy decisions to Congress. His administration successfully neutralized special interest groups (eg, medical device makers, the pharmaceutical industry, and health insurance plans) by bringing them to the table to negotiate. They managed to attract public support by emphasizing that insured Americans could keep their existing coverage.[9,10] Ultimately, in March, 2010, against long odds, the landmark Patient Protection and Affordable Care Act

Conflicts of interest: None.
Grant Support: This research was supported, in part, by a career development award from the National Institutes of Health (K12HS019468).
Division of Gastroenterology and Hepatology, University of North Carolina School of Medicine, CB 7080, Chapel Hill, NC 27599, USA
E-mail address: sdorn@med.unc.edu

(PPACA) was signed into law. Soon, PPACA was amended by the Health Care and Education Reconciliation Act and the result was a large collection of patchwork-style reforms that build on the existing health care system.[9,10] Most notably, it expanded coverage to approximately 30 million American citizens who were previously uninsured. Secondarily, it changed financial incentives and altered flow of information in ways designed to improve quality and slow the rate of cost growth.[11] In this article the elements of reform most relevant to clinical gastroenterology are reviewed, the ongoing challenges that this legislation faces are discussed, and the potential implications for clinical practice are considered.

EXPANDED HEALTH INSURANCE COVERAGE

PPACA uses a combination of subsidies, mandates, regulations, and public and private insurance expansions to extend health insurance to most (but not all) of the more than 50 million[2] currently uninsured Americans. Already the bill has established high risk-pools for uninsured individuals with preexisting conditions, extended coverage to children on their parents' insurance up to age 26 years, and offered credits to small businesses that choose to offer insurance to their employees.

By 2014 a mandate will require that all citizens have and all large businesses (50 or more employees) offer qualifying health insurance or face financial penalties. Qualifying criteria for Medicaid and the Children's Health Insurance Plan (CHIP) will be expanded. Many of those who do not qualify for these programs (or their employers) will be given subsidies to purchase insurance on health insurance exchanges, which essentially are an "analog to farmers' markets on which competing insurers offer their products, subject to a set of regulations that make transactions in the marketplace transparent and honorable, and the competition among insurers fair."[12] Despite these efforts, the Centers for Medicare and Medicaid Services (CMS) actuary estimates that by 2019 23 million citizens will remain uninsured,[13] as will all undocumented immigrants.

PPACA also imposes new regulations on the private insurance industry. It creates minimum standards for coverage, eliminates exclusions because of preexisting illnesses, removes annual and lifetime dollar limits on essential benefits, ends the practice of rescinding coverage because of illness, limits medical loss ratios (defined as the proportion of premium dollars spent on administrative costs and profits), and restricts the upper and lower range of insurance premium costs from varying for any reason other than age, family size, geographic region, and tobacco use. There also are provisions designed to simplify administrative processes for both beneficiaries and providers. For instance, insurers will be required to post on their Web site whether particular tests are covered, how much it will reimburse, and how much patients will have to pay.

Particularly relevant to gastroenterologists is Section 2713, which states that Medicare, Medicaid, and all new commercial insurance plans "shall not impose any cost sharing requirements for evidence-based items or services that have in effect a rating of 'A' or 'B' in the current recommendations of the United States Preventive Services Task Force." This will eliminate deductible payments, copayments, and coinsurance for several colon cancer screening modalities, including screening colonoscopy. However, because of the technical language of the bill, the waiver will not cover copayments for diagnostic and therapeutic procedures, including screening colonoscopies during which a polypectomy is performed. It is also unclear whether insurers will apply cost-sharing waivers to surveillance colonoscopy. Rectifying these issues will require a legislative fix, although this is unlikely given the current political climate.

CHANGING INCENTIVES

According to former CMS Administrator Mark McClellan, "The way Medicare pays physicians and health professionals is the linchpin for real reform because of the importance of physician decisions in overall health care quality and cost."[14] Over the short-term the currently dominant fee-for-service (FFS) model is preserved, although PPACA requires revaluation of certain procedure codes, and extends pay for quality reporting and value-based purchasing initiatives. Over the longer-term, PPACA sets in place a series of efforts designed to shift payment toward broader units of service.

FFS Under PPACA

Over the short-term most physicians will continue to be paid under the FFS model. FFS reimburses physicians for discrete services rendered. Through an intricate process of time and intensity analysis based on surveys of practitioners and cross-walking with like procedures, each service is assigned several relative value units (RVUs) on the Medicare Resource Based Relative Value Scale fee schedule,[15] which guides reimbursement for all Medicare plans as well as most Medicaid and private insurance plans.[16] The number of RVUs is equal to the weighted sum of the estimated amount of physician work (W) (52% of RVU), practice expenses (PE) (44% of RVU), and malpractice costs (MP) (4% of RVU) required to furnish a service, each of which is adjusted based on geographic location (Geographic Practice Cost Index [GPCI]). Next, RVUs are multiplied by a conversion factor (CF) to determine actual dollar payments.

$$\text{Payment} = [(\text{W RVU} \times \text{W GPCI}) + (\text{PE RVU} \times \text{PE GPCI}) + (\text{MP RVU} \times \text{MP GPCI})] \times \text{CF}$$

The CF is determined through the controversial sustainable growth rate (SGR) mechanism. The SGR, which was enacted in 1998 to contain Medicare Part B spending, compares spending with a target benchmark that is based primarily on growth in the overall economy, as well as estimates of medical inflation, and growth in the number of Medicare beneficiaries.[17] If spending is less than targeted the CF is adjusted upwards. Conversely, if actual spending exceeds targeted spending the CF is adjusted downwards and payments are cut, unless Congress intervenes.

Despite noble intentions, the SGR is fundamentally flawed because it attempts to restrict spending solely by limiting physician payment rates without accounting for ongoing growth in the volume and complexity of health care services.[18] In addition, because the SGR mechanism aggregates spending across all physicians, it does not provide any incentive for individual physicians to control cost growth.[19] Each year the volume of health care services continues to increase and, consequently, health care spending continues to outpace overall economic growth. In turn, each year the SGR calls for downward adjustments to the CF and, by extension, cuts in physician payment. However, the mere mention of reduced Medicare payments reflexively triggers alarm in the elderly community, concerned that they will lose access to care. Afraid to alienate this important constituency, each year (since 2003) Congress has passed last-minute legislative fixes that avert payment cuts, although leaving the SGR otherwise intact.[20] However, because spending targets are cumulative (ie, last year's expenditure target * SGR = current year's expenditure target), spending that exceeds the target one year accumulates in future years until it is recouped.[21] Other legislative imperatives make payment of this accumulating debt mandatory so it cannot be ignored from a fiscal perspective. Thus, these short-term legislative fixes have made the long-term solution more expensive.[22] For instance, in 2012 physicians face a 30% reduction.[19]

PPACA did not address the SGR mechanism, primarily because doing so would have added $210 billion to the price tag of the bill.[23] Over the long-term this situation leaves physicians (particularly those who are procedural based, such as gastroenterologists) vulnerable to massive payment cuts. The Medicare Payment Advisory Commission, the Congressional agency that advises Congress on issues pertaining to Medicare, stated that "Replacing the SGR and expenditure targets with a different payment structure – without the current scheduled cuts – presents an opportunity to introduce needed payment reforms. That is, in exchange for eliminating the future fee cuts, reforms could be made in FFS Medicare to improve the accuracy of payments under the physician fee schedule, to increase payments for cognitive (or nonprocedural) services relative to procedural services, and to give the Secretary discretion to adjust payments."[19]

Although PPACA largely preserved the FFS model in the short-term, and did not address the SGR mechanism, it did implement 2 main changes to the FFS system. First, PPACA assumes $200 billion can be saved by tying Medicare market-basket payment updates to productivity gains in the rest of the private sector economy. Because health care providers are unlikely to be able to increase their productivity enough (ie, to the same degree as firms in the private economy at large) to offset these reduced payments, the result will be shrinking (and possibly negative) Medicare profit margins. In turn, providers will likely threaten to stop accepting Medicare patients unless Congress intervenes.[13,24]

Gastroenterologists are more likely to be affected by the second main change to FFS, codified in PPACA Section 3134, which instructs the Secretary of Health and Human Services (HHS) to "periodically identify services as potentially misvalued … and review [them] and make appropriate adjustments." Scrutiny will be directed toward codes for which there has been the fastest growth or substantial changes in practice expenses, as well as codes for recently established technologies, and those that have not been subject to review since implementation of the RVU system. Based on these criteria, 4 endoscopy codes are slated for review in 2011: Current Procedural Terminology (CPT) codes 43235 (upper gastrointestinal endoscopy), 43239 (upper gastrointestinal endoscopy with biopsy), 45380 (colonoscopy with biopsy), and 45385 (colonoscopy with removal of lesion by snare technique). For each of these procedures the Secretary will conduct surveys, collect data, and perform analyses to determine whether and how to adjust the amount of work these services require (which, as stated earlier, accounts for 52% of the RVU). This adjustment will be largely determined by the amount of time it takes to perform a service (intraservice time), as well as the preservice and postservice time.[25] Because time estimates previously used to determine work requirements for these procedures (**Table 1**) are likely less than real-world time requirements, gastroenterologists will probably see reduced Medicare reimbursement for these procedures.

Quality Reporting

A series of laws passed between 2006 and 2008 (including the Tax Relief and Health Care Act, The Medicare, Medicaid, and SCHIP Extension Act of 2007, and the Medicare Improvements for Patients and Providers Act of 2008) established the Physician Quality Reporting Initiative (PQRI), which offered bonus payments to providers who reported performance on select quality measures. For gastroenterologists the choice of measures was limited to those related to treatment and management of hepatitis C (measures 84–87, 89–90, and 183–184) and several related to gastroesophageal reflux

Table 1					
Time estimates previously used to determine relative value of select endoscopic procedures					
CPT	Descriptor	Preservice (min)	Intraservice (min)	Postservice (min)	Total (min)
43235	Upper endoscopy	18	20	25	63
43239	Upper endoscopy with biopsy	27	34	23.5	84.5
45380	Colonoscopy with biopsy	45	51.5	22	118.5
45385	Colonoscopy with snare polypectomy	16	43	15	74

Data from CMS. Physician Time File. Available at: http://www.cms.gov/apps/ama/license.asp?file=/physicianfeesched/downloads/phy_time_file.zip.

(subsequently deleted from the measure set). A colorectal cancer screening measure was included, but was used mostly by primary care providers (measure 113). Later measure 185 (colonoscopy interval for patients with a history of adenomatous polyps–avoidance of inappropriate use) was added. In 2009 only 866 gastroenterologists (15% of those eligible) participated in PQRI. Participants earned, on average, $2635 (range $3–$13,842) in bonuses.[26] PPACA made several changes to the program that should encourage more gastroenterologists to participate. Most visibly, recognizing that it is no longer an initiative, PQRI was renamed the Physician Quality Reporting System (PQRS). In addition, PPACA extends pay-for-reporting bonus payments to 2014; physicians who report quality data using Medicare Part B claims, a qualified PQRS registry, or a qualified electronic health record (EHR) will receive a 0.5% bonus. Starting in 2015 the carrot is swapped for a stick; physicians who do not participate will be subject to 1.5% (2% in 2016 and beyond) cuts in Medicare reimbursement.

Value-based Purchasing

Value-based purchasing programs offer financial incentives to providers who deliver demonstrably high-value care, defined as "high benefits of services in relation to their cost."[27] CMS views "value-based purchasing as an important step to revamping how Medicare pays for health care services, moving the program toward rewarding better value, outcomes, and innovations, instead of merely volume."[28] In this vein, PPACA extends Medicare value-based payment programs to physicians, hospitals, and ambulatory surgery centers (ASCs).

For physicians, by 2017 Medicare FFS payments will be adjusted based on a value-based payment modifier that reflects the quality and cost of the care that they provide. Higher-value providers will receive across-the-board bonuses, whereas low-value providers will be penalized. Defining quality and cost of care is both theoretically and practically difficult.[29] CMS pledges to use transparent methods and work with physicians to develop composite, risk-adjusted quality and cost measures that can then be used as payment modifiers.[30] It will publish the initial set of these measures by January 1, 2012.

CMS will also soon extend value-based purchasing to hospitals. Between 2013 and 2017 hospital reimbursement for all Diagnostic Related Groups under the prospective payment system will be gradually cut from 1% to 2%. Hospitals will then be given a chance to earn back reduced revenue through value-based bonuses. These bonuses will be determined by performance on a set of yet-to-be-decided composite measures that will blend quality, efficiency, and patient experience metrics for select conditions (initially these will include myocardial infarction, congestive heart failure, and pneumonia, as well as certain surgical procedures).

PPACA also requires CMS to extend value-based purchasing to ASCs. As outlined in a recently released roadmap, CMS intends to use "reliable and straightforward scoring methodologies" to compare ASC performance on a set of nationally endorsed measures with both national benchmarks and past performance. Higher-performing centers will receive increased Medicare payments, which, given budget-neutrality requirements, will likely come at the expense of their lower-performing counterparts.[28]

Bundled Payments

FFS has been vilified for encouraging quantity over quality, penalizing certain labor-intensive activities (eg, spending time talking with patients and coordinating care), favoring procedures over cognitive services, and ultimately fueling the fragmentation of care.[31] It also places physicians at financial risk when they try to undertake innovative ideas that may improve health and reduce use.[32] Consequently, many argue that radically new payment models are needed to improve quality and reducing costs.[33] To this end, PPACA established the CMS Innovation Center to develop, pilot test, and implement various novel payment models that shift reimbursement away from discrete services (ie, FFS) toward broader units of care.[30]

One such effort is using a single bundled payment that combines payments across multiple providers and settings, thereby encouraging providers to coordinate care and work together to reduce costs across all the services within a bundle. Mandatory quality metrics are also included to help ensure that efforts to reduce costs do not diminish quality. For instance, the Medicare Acute Care Episode demonstration project pays a fixed amount to both hospitals and physicians for all orthopedic and cardiac procedure related services, spanning both inpatient and outpatient settings. PPACA requires CMS to start implementing episode-based bundles for an initial set of conditions by 2013. Doing so will require overcoming major technical challenges, such as defining episodes of care, identifying appropriate quality measures, and negotiating single payments across multiple providers.[32] For the gastroenterologist, calculating appropriate reimbursement will require careful definition of what services fall within their responsibility vis-à-vis the primary care provider or other specialists. Such definitions have not yet been negotiated, much less embedded in payer databases.

Shared Savings and Accountable Care Organizations

The shared savings model is an alternative to bundled payments that circumvents the complexities of defining episodes of care (as is required for bundled payments), although it still creates incentives for providers to work together to deliver better care at lower costs. In this model, groups of providers who join together to deliver care are allowed to share savings achieved in overall per capita spending. Certain quality benchmarks are attached to shared savings to prevent merely skimping on care.

Shared savings models set the stage for accountable care organizations (ACOs), defined as integrated groups of providers who jointly assume responsibility for the cost and quality of all care delivered to a defined population. PPACA Section 3022 established ACOs as a permanent program (rather than a pilot program) that will take effect by January 1, 2012. Although the legislation flexibly allows ACO providers to assume various organizational forms (including integrated delivery systems, multi-specialty group practices, physician hospital organizations, and independent practice associations[34]), it requires that they have formal legal, leadership, and management structures, care for at least 5000 Medicare beneficiaries, fulfill certain patient-centeredness criteria, use defined processes to measure and report quality and cost data, promote evidenced-based medicine, and coordinate care.

ACOs may be paid under several variations of the shared savings model. The asymmetric (also known as 1-sided risk) shared savings model continues to reimburse ACOs' FFS payments for each service delivered, and offers a bonus to those ACOs that spend less than their target and meet quality requirements.[35] Alternatively, the symmetric (also known as 2-sided risk) savings model allows ACOs to share a greater proportion of cost savings, as long as they are willing to risk penalties for spending more than the target. The desire to avoid penalties and to reap rewards creates a double incentive to save, and therefore symmetric models may more effectively limit costs.[36] Further along the spectrum is partial capitation, which mixes limited FFS payments with prospective lump-sum payments that are made regardless of use, thereby putting ACOs at the greatest financial risk, although allowing for the greatest possible rewards.[37,38]

From the start, critics have argued that considerable organizational, cultural, and legal barriers will make forming ACOs challenging. Others have questioned whether ACOs can save costs. For instance, in the Physician Group Practice Demonstration project, which served as an early ACO model, only 5 of the 10 already integrated practices achieved cost savings, which, on subsequent analysis, may have been more the result of previous cost trends than changes in care delivery.[39]

Criticism toward ACOs grew sharper on March 31, 2011 after the Secretary of HHS released a set of ACO draft regulations. Among other things, various provider groups, hospitals, and professional associations complained that the limited available savings (which would be based on historical costs, thereby making it more difficult for already efficient ACOs to generate savings) would not justify the considerable ACO start-up costs, and that quality reporting requirements were too burdensome (ACOs would be required to measure and report 65 quality measures).[40,41] The American Medical Group Association (AMGA) commented that the draft rule is "overly prescriptive, operationally burdensome, and the incentives are too difficult to achieve....[and that] 93% of AMGA members would not enroll as an ACO under the current regulatory framework."[42] At the time of this writing, the draft regulations are undergoing revision. The final ruling will strongly determine the fate of ACOs.

Independent Payment Advisory Board

A key PPACA mechanism for controlling cost growth is the Independent Payment Advisory Board (IPAB), a 15 member nonpartisan board tasked with presenting Congress with comprehensive proposals for holding Medicare spending at or less than targeted levels. Starting in 2015 the target is set to the general rate of health care inflation. By 2019 the target resets to percent change in the gross domestic product plus 1 percentage point. If Medicare growth exceeds these targets (which, based on historical trends[43] seems nearly certain) then IPAB must formulate a set of recommendations to reduce spending. These recommendations cannot include anything that rations care, raises taxes, increases premiums, or changes benefits. However, IPAB can recommend reducing physician payments. Congress must then consider IPAB's recommendation and either approve it through a vote or devise a suitable alternative. If no legislation is passed then the IPAB recommendations are automatically sent to the Secretary of HHS who is required to implement them. Not surprisingly, IPAB has been one of the most controversial PPACA provisions. Its full impact (and fate) will be determined by ongoing political challenges.[44]

IMPROVING INFORMATION

In addition to expanding coverage and redesigning incentives to improve care, recent health care reform legislation seeks to improve the quality, management, and flow of information. In turn, this legislation should enhance decision making, improve coordination of care, and reduce waste.

HIT

HIT, which includes EHRs, computerized order entry, and electronic prescribing, has been touted as a means for building a safer, more effective, and more efficient health care system.[45] Nonetheless, physicians and hospitals have been slow to adopt EHRs.[46] Accordingly, as part of the 2009 stimulus bill (American Recovery and Reinvestment Act), the Health Information Technology for Economic and Clinical Health Act established incentive payments and grant programs for speeding the adoption and meaningful use of certified EHRs.

CMS has since defined an evolving, 3-stage set of criteria for defining meaningful use. Stage 1 mainly revolves around electronic data capture. Providers will be required to electronically record key parts of a patient's history (demographics, vitals, active medication/problem lists, smoking), electronically prescribe, create care-summary documents for patients, implement at least 1 decision support tool, and report clinical quality. Stages 2 and 3 will focus on exchange of electronic data and will use more stringent requirements.[47]

Eligible professionals (including gastroenterologists who participate in Medicare or Medicaid and provide at least 90% of their services outside the inpatient setting) who show meaningful use (based on reaching a preset threshold on a set of functionality and clinical quality measures) will receive bonus payments (which cannot exceed 75% of annual Medicare charges) for up to 5 years from either Medicare or Medicaid, not both. These payments are front loaded; those who meet meaningful use by 2012 can receive $44,000 in Medicare incentives, whereas those who wait until 2014 will receive only $24,000. Meanwhile, providers who do not meet meaningful use by 2015 face a 1% reduction in Medicare payments, which, by 2018, will reach 5%.[48]

There is a related initiative to spur electronic prescribing. Physicians who use qualified e-prescription systems to prescribe for at least 10% of Medicare encounters are entitled to 1% bonus (although not if they also receive meaningful use bonuses). Similar to PQRS and meaningful use, by 2013 this incentive payment will be phased out and penalties will be levied on those who do not e-prescribe.

Quality Reporting Programs

PPACA requires reporting quality data collected for PQRS, meaningful use, and other purposes to consumers on the Physician Compare CMS Web site. In theory, consumers will then use this information to identify high-value providers. In addition, CMS will be required to create provider feedback reports that will compare a provider's pattern of resource use (most likely overall per capita cost) and quality (on a core of 12 process measures) to that achieved by their peer group. To create these reports, CMS will first need to develop methodologies for attributing costs/quality to specific providers; determining minimum sample size requirements, adjusting results for baseline patient characteristics, and identifying suitable comparison peer groups.

CER

CER analyzes the impact of different diagnostic and treatment options. The results may be used by patients and providers to choose diagnostic tests and therapies that achieve better, more efficient results. In turn, this strategy may generate considerable cost savings.[49] The 2009 stimulus bill included a $1.1 billion investment into to CER. PPACA later extended this investment by establishing the Patient-Centered Outcomes Research Institute (PCORI), which it funds with nearly $500 million each year. However, given widespread fear that CER will lead to rationing and cookbook medicine, PPACA specifically states that PCORI cannot be used to conduct cost-effectiveness analysis (a subset of CER "that examines the comparative impact of expenditures on different health interventions"[50]) and PCORI study results cannot be used to deny coverage for any services.[51] Consequently, potential savings from this nonbinding research will likely be small.[13]

WHAT COMES NEXT?

Even with landmark legislation signed into law, health care reform is not a fait accompli. Aaron and Reischauer[52] wrote, "Far from having ended, the war to make health care reform an enduring success has just begun. Winning that war will require administrative determination and imagination and as much political resolve as was needed to pass the legislation."

Rulemaking Process

Administrative agencies are delegated power by Congress to act as agents for the Executive and promulgate regulations designed to carry out Congress's intent. In turn, Congress maintains a variable level of control over the rulemaking process by determining the nature of the regulations (ie, whether the regulations must be implemented by a particular date, include certain substantive elements, or follow certain procedures), and by controlling agency appropriations, writing letters to agency officials, and conducting oversight and confirmation hearings. Meanwhile, lobbyists continually fight to secure interpretations of the law that are favorable to the stakeholders they represent.

PPACA gives various agencies (most notably the Department of HHS) considerable authority to create the regulations that will fill in the details of the legislation. Some sections of PPACA require new regulations, some permit new regulations at the discretion of the agencies, and others relate to existing rules.[53] For instance, whereas PPACA set a broad framework for ACOs, CMS regulations will determine how ACOs operate.

Political, Legal, and Budgetary Challenges

In the face of mounting and unsustainable federal and state deficits,[1] as well as the most polarized Congress in recent history,[54] health care reform has become as a proxy in a larger battle over the fundamental role of government.[55] Democrats argue that we cannot afford to not reform health care and, as outlined in PPACA, favor using a top-down approach to controlling health care costs, such as the CMS Innovation Center and IPAB. Conversely, Republicans argue that health care can be best improved using a decentralization approach, such as managed competition through which consumers are given premium support (albeit at lower amounts than in PPACA) and allowed greater choice in choosing a health plan and provider.[55,56]

This battle is being fought on many fronts, perhaps most visibly the courts. At the time of this writing there are 26 federal lawsuits that seek to overturn PPACA on numerous grounds, the most serious being whether Congress has the authority to mandate that individuals obtain insurance. This situation will likely come down to whether the Supreme Court considers the mandate to be a form of economic regulation (which would justify Congress under its power to regulate interstate commerce) and whether the fine for not obtaining insurance is considered a tax (which would justify Congress under its taxing powers) or a penalty.[57,58]

The battle is also being waged in federal and state legislatures. Opponents of health care reform are trying to deny agencies funding to carry out those PPACA directives that require Congressional appropriations, including $50 million for medical malpractice reform demonstration projects, as well as other projects to develop quality measure and improve health care coordination.[59] Likewise, several state governments have passed legislation that attempts to nullify certain provisions of PPACA.

And soon the fate of health care reform may be decided by election polls. The challenge for health care reform survival is that the reform bill lacks an identity ("PPACA" does not exactly roll off the tongue) and, given that insurance coverage will not be appreciably expanded until 2014, most Americans do not understand how this complex legislation may improve their lives. Changes in political leadership from elections in 2012 could lead to repeal or, more likely, substantive modification of the law.[60] However, if PPACA survives lawsuits and political resistance, then over time its prospects will start to increase, just as social security and Medicare have become indispensable to most American families.[10]

Impact on Gastroenterology?

With so many variables it is difficult to precisely predict the impact that health reform will have on gastroenterology, but several tends seem to be likely as follows:

1. *Demand for gastroenterology services will increase.* The Chief Actuary for CMS estimates that PPACA will extend coverage to an additional 34 million Americans,[13] some of whom may have existing digestive disorders and others who are more than 50 years old. However, more than half of the newly insured will be covered by Medicaid, which, on average, reimburses at only two-thirds Medicare rates.[61] Will gastroenterologists be able to treat these newly insured patients?[62] Either way, eliminating out-of-pocket expenses should increase screening colonoscopy use, although this will provide less incentive for patients to choose low cost locals (ASCs for example) for their endoscopic procedures.

2. *Gastroenterologist salaries will decrease.* In 2010 the median salary for gastroenterologists was $463,995, more than double that of primary care physicians.[63] PPACA promises to shrink this specialist-generalist pay gap.[64] Primary care physicians will receive 10% bonuses from Medicare, and Medicaid payments will be brought up to match these new Medicare levels.[30] Meanwhile, gastroenterologists will almost certainly see payment cuts once certain key procedure codes are revaluated. Furthermore, without legislative intervention ASC facility fees will continue to decrease, and because the ASC value-based payment program will be budget neutral, bonuses for some groups will occur at the expense of others. Over the long-term, movement away from FFS will shift financial risk to gastroenterologists and other physicians.[56] Meanwhile, gastroenterologists and other physicians will remain especially vulnerable to the unresolved SGR mechanism, as well as the ability of IPAB to recommend physician payment cuts.

3. *There will be an increased administrative burden.* Practicing physicians will become even more laden with administrative tasks. They will be required to install and meaningfully use EHRs, prescribe electronically, and better coordinate care with

their colleagues. Various programs (including meaningful use, PQRS, value-based purchasing programs, and bundled payments) will require gastroenterologists to measure and report their performance on various metrics. Ultimately, productivity and physician satisfaction may decrease.

Traditionally, only hospitals have been able to invest in HIT and management to the extent that PPACA requires. Thus, many gastroenterologists may retire or sell their practices to hospital-dominated, vertically integrated health care systems.[11] Others may attempt to pool resources and gain a modicum of negotiating leverage by partnering with competitors to form either loose alliances or horizontally integrated supergroups with dozens, if not hundreds, of gastroenterology providers. Whatever the ultimate outcome, 1 thing is for certain: health care reform is changing the face of clinical gastroenterology.

REFERENCES

1. The National Commission on Fiscal Responsibility and Reform. 2010. The Moment of Truth. Available at: http://www.fiscalcommission.gov/sites/fiscalcommission.gov/files/documents/TheMomentofTruth12_1_2010.pdf. Accessed January 3, 2011.
2. The Uninsured: A Primer. Key Facts About Americans Without Health Insurance. Menlo Park (CA): Kaiser Family Foundation; 2010. Available at: http://www.kff.org/uninsured/upload/7451-06.pdf. Accessed June 5, 2011.
3. Institute of Medicine. Committee on Quality of Health Care in America. Crossing the quality chasm: a new health system for the 21st century. Washington, DC: National Academy Press; 2001.
4. Davis K, Schoen C, Schoenbaum SC, et al. Mirror, mirror on the wall: an international update on the comparative performance of American health care. New York: The Commonwealth Fund; 2007.
5. Starr P. The social transformation of American medicine. New York: Basic Books; 1982.
6. Blumenthal D, Monroe J. The heart of power: health and politics in the oval office. Berkley and Los Angeles, CA: University of California Press; 2009.
7. Oberlander J. Presidential politics and the resurgence of health care reform. N Engl J Med 2007;357:2101–4.
8. The American Recovery and Reinvestment Act HR, P.L. 111-5, 123 Stat 115. February 19, 2009.
9. Oberlander J. Long time coming: why health reform finally passed. Health Aff (Millwood) 2010;29:1112–6.
10. Jacobs LR, Skocpol T. Health care reform and American politics. New York: Oxford University Press; 2010.
11. Kocher R, Emanuel EJ, DeParle NA. The Affordable Care Act and the future of clinical medicine: the opportunities and challenges. Ann Intern Med 2010;153:536–9.
12. Reinhardt U. Defining 'Health Care Reform'. New York: The New York Times; 2009.
13. Foster RS. Estimated financial effects of the "Patient Protection and Affordable Care Act," as amended. Baltimore (MD): Centers for Medicare and Medicaid Services; 2010.
14. McClellan MB. Next steps on Medicare reform now. Available at: http://www.brookings.edu/opinions/2011/0520_medicare_reform_mcclellan.aspx. Accessed May 21, 2011.

15. Ginsburg PB, Berenson RA. Revising Medicare's physician fee schedule–much activity, little change. N Engl J Med 2007;356:1201–3.
16. Smith SL, Eagle R, Klemp T. Coding and Medical Information Group, American Medical Association. Medicare RBRVS: The Physicians' Guide, 2006. Chicago: American Medical Association; 2006.
17. The sustainable growth rate formula for setting Medicare's physician payment rates. Washington, DC: Congressional Budget Office; 2006.
18. Aaron HJ. The SGR for physician payment–an indispensable abomination. N Engl J Med 2010;363:403–5.
19. Report to the Congress: Medicare and the health care delivery system. Washington, DC: MEDPAC; 2011.
20. Wilk S, Phillips RL Jr. Medicare's (un)sustainable growth rate. Fam Pract Manag 2008;15:9–10.
21. CMS Report 4 - A-05 Report of the Council on Medical Service. Washington, DC: Centers for Medicare and Medicaid Services; 2005.
22. Wilensky GR. Reforming Medicare's physician payment system. N Engl J Med 2009;360:653–5.
23. H.R. 3961. Medicare Physician Payment Reform Act of 2009. Congressional Budget Office; 2009. Available at: http://www.cbo.gov/ftpdocs/107xx/doc10704/hr3961.pdf. Accessed June 1, 2011.
24. Berenson RA. Implementing health care reform–why Medicare matters. N Engl J Med 2010;363:101–3.
25. Mabry CD, McCann BC, Harris JA, et al. The use of intraservice work per unit of time (IWPUT) and the building block method (BBM) for the calculation of surgical work. Ann Surg 2005;241:929–38 [discussion: 938–40].
26. Centers for Medicare and Medicaid Services. Physician Quality Reporting System. 2009 Reporting Experience Including Trends. Available at: http://www.cms.gov/PQRS. Accessed June 1, 2011.
27. Tompkins CP, Higgins AR, Ritter GA. Measuring outcomes and efficiency in Medicare value-based purchasing. Health Aff (Millwood) 2009;28:w251–61.
28. Report to Congress: Medicare ambulatory surgical center value-based purchasing implementation plan. New York: US Department of Health and Human Services; 2011.
29. Dorn SD. Gastroenterology in a new era of accountability: Part 1–an overview of performance measurement. Clin Gastroenterol Hepatol 2011;9:563–6.
30. Ginsburg PB. Rapidly evolving physician-payment policy–more than the SGR. N Engl J Med 2011;364:172–6.
31. Miller HD. Creating payment systems to accelerate value-driven health care: issues and options for policy reform. New York: The Commonwealth Fund; 2007.
32. McClellan M. Reforming payments to healthcare providers: the key to slowing healthcare cost growth while improving quality? J Econ Perspect 2011;25:69–92.
33. Tollen LA, Fund C. Physician organization in relation to quality and efficiency of care: a synthesis of recent literature. New York: The Commonwealth Fund; 2008.
34. Shortell SM, Casalino LP, Fisher ES. Achieving the vision: structural change. In: Crosson FJ, Tollen LA, editors. Partners in health: how physicians and hospitals can be accountable together. San Francisco (CA): Jossey-Bass; 2010.
35. Berenson RA. Shared Savings Program for accountable care organizations: a bridge to nowhere? Am J Manag Care 2010;16:721–6.
36. Hackbarth GM. MEDPAC letter to CMS. November 22, 2010. Available at: http://www.medpac.gov/documents/11222010_ACO_COMMENT_MedPAC.pdf. Accessed August 19, 2011.

37. McClellan M, McKethan AN, Lewis JL, et al. A national strategy to put account-able care into practice. Health Aff (Millwood) 2010;29:982–90.
38. Dorn SD. Gastroenterology in a new era of accountability: part 3–accountable care organizations. Clin Gastroenterol Hepatol 2011;9:750–3.
39. Iglehart JK. Assessing an ACO prototype–Medicare's Physician Group Practice demonstration. N Engl J Med 2010;364(3):198–200.
40. Ginsburg PB. Spending to save–ACOs and the Medicare Shared Savings Program. N Engl J Med 2011;364:2085–6.
41. Iglehart JK. The ACO regulations–some answers, more questions. N Engl J Med 2011;364:e35.
42. American Medical Group Association. Letter to Donald M. Berwick re: Medicare Shared Savings Program: Accountable Care Organizations. Available at: http://www.amga.org/advocacy/MGAC/Letters/05112011.pdf. Accessed June 1, 2011.
43. Boccuti C, Moon M. Comparing Medicare and private insurers: growth rates in spending over three decades. Health Aff (Millwood) 2003;22:230–7.
44. Aaron HJ. The Independent Payment Advisory Board–Congress's"Good Deed". N Engl J Med 2011;364(25):2377–9.
45. Shekelle PG, Morton SC, Keeler EB. Costs and benefits of health information technology. Evid Rep Technol Assess (Full Rep) 2006;132:1–71.
46. DesRoches CM, Campbell EG, Rao SR, et al. Electronic health records in ambu-latory care–a national survey of physicians. N Engl J Med 2008;359:50–60.
47. Jha AK. Meaningful use of electronic health records: the road ahead. JAMA 2010; 304:1709–10.
48. Blumenthal D, Tavenner M. The "meaningful use" regulation for electronic health records. N Engl J Med 2010;363:501–4.
49. Orszag PR. Research on the comparative effectiveness of medical treatments: issues and options for an expanded federal role. Washington, DC: Congressional Budget Office; 2007.
50. Gold MR, Siegel JE, Russell LB, et al. Cost-effectiveness in health and medicine. New York: Oxford University Press; 1996.
51. Kamerow D. PCORI: odd name, important job, potential trouble. BMJ 2011;342: d2635.
52. Aaron HJ, Reischauer RD. The war isn't over. N Engl J Med 2010;362:1259–61.
53. Copeland CW. Rulemaking requirements and authorities in the Patient Protection and Affordable Care Act (PPACA). Washington, DC: US Congressional Research Service; 2011. p. R41180.
54. Brownstein R. Pulling Apart. National Journal. National Journal; 2011. Available at: http://www.nationaljournal.com/magazine/congress-hits-new-peak-in-polarization-20110224?page=1. Accessed June 1, 2011.
55. Brooks D. Where wisdom lives. New York: The New York Times; 2011.
56. Jost TS. Consensus and conflict in health system reform–the Republican budget plan and the ACA. N Engl J Med 2011;364:e40.
57. Balkin JM. The constitutionality of the individual mandate for health insurance. N Engl J Med 2010;362:482–3.
58. Chaikind H, Copeland CW, Redhead CS, et al. PPACA: a brief overview of the law, implementation, and legal challenges. Washington, DC: US Congressional Research Service; 2011. p. R41664.
59. Redhead CS. PPACA: appropriations and fund transfers in the Patient Protection and Affordable Care Act (PPACA). Washington, DC: US Congressional Research Service; 2011. p. R41301.

60. Marmor T, Oberlander J. The patchwork: health reform, American style. Soc Sci Med 2010;72:125–8.
61. Zuckerman S, Williams AF, Stockley KE. Trends in Medicaid physician fees, 2003–2008. Health Aff (Millwood) 2009;28:w510–9.
62. Zinberg JM. When patients call, will physicians respond? JAMA 2011;305: 2011–2.
63. Crane M. Physician Compensation and Production Survey - 2011 Report Based on 2010 Data. Medscape News; 2011. Available at: http://www.medscape.com/viewarticle/744645. Accessed June 19, 2011.
64. Bodenheimer T, Matin M, Yoshio Laing B. The specialist-generalist income gap: can we narrow it? J Gen Intern Med 2008;23:1539–41.

Impact of Health Care Reform on the Independent GI Practice

Klaus Mergener, MD, PhD, MBA

KEYWORDS

- Health care • Reform • Gastroenterology • Endoscopy
- Private practice • Independent practice
- Patient Protection and Affordable Care Act (PPACA)
- Affordable Care Act (ACA)

"When nothing is sure, everything is possible"
—[Dame Margaret Drabble, English Novelist, born 1939]

It has been widely recognized that the United States health care system is expensive, fragmented, and ineffective. According to the latest data set from the Organization for Economic Development (OECD), health care expenditures are outpacing overall economic productivity by 2% annually and now account for 17.3% of gross domestic product.[1] The United States currently spends a total of $2.5 trillion per year on health care, or approximately $8000 per person, 2.5 times more than the average developed nation.[2,3] Despite such massive spending, the United States is alone among developed countries in not providing health care coverage for all its citizens, and is being ranked last or second to last in quality, access, patient safety, efficiency, adoption of information technology, and quality improvement, when compared with Australia, Canada, Germany, New Zealand, and the United Kingdom.[4,5] With government budgets increasingly dominated by the need to finance the cost of Medicare and Medicaid, and the country's competitive position in a global market eroding, the political pressure has been rising to fix what is perceived to be a broken system. The health reform law now commonly referred to as the Accountable Care Act (ACA) of 2010 is the most comprehensive effort yet to accomplish this task.

Many have opined that the fragmentation of the health care system, the lack of care coordination between sites of care and providers, as well as a payment system that incentivizes providers to maximize the volume of services, not the value of care,

Conflicts of interest: Cofounder, U.S. Gastro, LLC.
Digestive Health Specialists, Gastroenterology, MultiCare Health System, 3209 South 23rd Street, Suite #340, Tacoma, WA 98415, USA
E-mail address: klausmergener@aol.com

are among the fundamental structural issues that need to be addressed. Berwick and colleagues[6] have proposed the "Triple Aim" as a conceptual framework for health reform, describing a set of interdependent goals that need to be pursued simultaneously to achieve high-value health care: improving the individual experience of care; improving the health of populations; and reducing the per capita cost of care of populations. Of importance, these investigators suggest care integration as the main vehicle for achieving the Triple Aim. The physician and writer Atul Gawande noted in his recent commencement address at Harvard Medical School that the complexity of medicine now exceeds the capabilities of individual physicians, and that the current structure of the health care system needs to be changed because it "emerged in an era when doctors could hold all the key information patients needed in their heads and manage everything required themselves."[7] Gawande further notes that in 1970, it took 2.5 full-time equivalents (FTEs) to take care of a typical hospital patient when today, due to the increasing complexity of medicine, that number has risen to more than 19 FTEs. He concludes that the complexity and range of required specialized skills force teamwork and well-tested protocols. Providers need to work more as "pit crews" and less as "cowboys," that is, system changes are necessary that encourage better communication and coordination between providers as well as transparency in measuring and rewarding quality performance. Therefore, while the need to reform the health care system has been long recognized and many efforts have been made, the recent passage of the ACA promises to accelerate this evolution with a specific emphasis on care integration, transparency in the pursuit of quality care, and accountability for and management of shared financial incentives.

CURRENT STATE OF GASTROENTEROLOGY PRACTICE

Before discussing the transformative impact of health care reform on gastroenterology (GI) practices, it is useful to take stock of the current state of GI in this country. Our specialty stands out among internal medicine specialties for its large proportion of ambulatory care and its procedure orientation. Gastroenterologists typically spend most of their time in ambulatory endoscopy units and in the office, focusing on colorectal and esophageal cancer prevention and on patients with a variety of prevalent disorders such as gastroesophageal reflux disease, liver problems, and inflammatory bowel disease. GI is a mostly consultative specialty, and as such is dependent on referrals from primary care providers. American medicine traditionally has been a "cottage industry" with most medical care being provided in small, privately owned practices. GI is no exception. According to recent surveys by the American Gastroenterological Association (AGA) and the American Society for Gastrointestinal Endoscopy (ASGE), approximately 80% of the 11,000 clinical gastroenterologists in the United States are practicing outside of academic medical centers.[3] (John Allen, AGA membership survey 2010, personal communication.) There has been a slow trend toward practice consolidation, but as of 2009 at least 50% to 60% of GI practices still had 4 or fewer physicians, and fewer than 20% had 11 or more physicians. Roughly half of private-practice gastroenterologists have a financial interest in an ambulatory endoscopy center (AEC). Informal estimates suggest that in 2012, approximately 65% to 70% of practice revenues are derived from procedures and related services. Although this makes GI practices uniquely vulnerable to disruptive technologies, at present endoscopy continues to be a key diagnostic tool and colonoscopy remains the preferred technique for colorectal cancer screening. Thus, any trends that put pressure on small practices or disproportionately affect procedure revenues will substantially alter the practice environment and pose potential threats to the financial stability of GI practitioners.[3]

GI practices have already encountered significant challenges in recent years related to escalating costs and a continued decline in reimbursement rates. As an example, the average Medicare physician payment for a colonoscopy with biopsy has steadily decreased from approximately $500 in 1989[8] to $265 in 2011. Practices have partially offset rising financial pressures by increasing efficiencies through optimizing endoscopy unit scheduling and workflow, adopting open-access endoscopy and GI hospitalist programs, and by adding ancillary service lines such as pathology, anesthesia, and infusion services. AECs are now "focus factories," providing much needed endoscopic services in a safe, efficient, reduced cost environment and in a patient-centered manner. However, the recent modification of the ambulatory surgical center payment system as put forth by the Centers for Medicare and Medicaid Services (CMS) has led to a precipitous decline in facility fees for endoscopic services (a decrease of more than 25% over 4 years) and has posed a significant threat to the viability of these centers.[9] Many AECs now operate at or below cost when performing a screening colonoscopy on a Medicare patient. In addition, GI practices are wrestling with an increasing number of unfunded regulatory mandates, the threat of further decreases in Medicare professional fees, the change in practice models of their primary care referral base, to name but a few ongoing challenges.

THE AFFORDABLE CARE ACT: GENERAL OBSERVATIONS

The Patient Protection and Affordable Care Act (Public Law 111-148)[10] was passed by the 111th United States Congress and signed by President Barack Obama March 23, 2010. Together with its subsequent amendment, the Health Care and Education Reconciliation Act of 2010 (Public Law 111-152),[11] this law is sometimes referred to as PPACA or simply as the Affordable Care Act (ACA). The ACA is an imposing piece of legislation which, on its 1083 pages, prescribes sweeping changes to the United States health care system to be implemented over several years. In general terms, the goals are to reform the insurance system, delivery system, and payment system for medical care in this country. To fully understand its impact, the ACA needs to be viewed in concert with other recent legislative efforts, such as the health information technology provisions of the American Recovery and Reinvestment Act (ARRA).[12] A detailed review of all aspects of the ACA is beyond the scope of this article, and the interested reader is referred to the article by Dorn elsewhere in this issue and other recent summaries.[13–15] Instead, the following discussion focuses on selected ACA provisions that are expected to result in trends that will transform GI care and the role of the independent GI practice in the delivery of such care.

It is worth noting that while the ACA provides an extensive legal framework, the specific effects of the reform on individual providers and practices will not be fully understood for several years. The "devil is in the details," and it is the implementation of the ACA, through regulations and interpretation of many provisions, that will ultimately determine many of these details. During the current multiyear implementation phase of the law, considerable uncertainty exists as to the exact shape of the health system in the postreform era, and providers who are currently trying to position themselves within the rapidly changing health care environment have to base their strategic decisions on "best-guess" scenarios. Physicians are generally risk averse, and it should therefore come as no surprise that some GI providers have decided to mitigate the risk associated with this period of uncertainty by "seeking shelter" with hospitals and health systems through selling practices and becoming employed providers. If previous economic pressures have put their practices on the fence, they believe that uncertainties associated with ACA are pushing them to give up their independent practice model. Whether this strategy will prove to be the best way forward will not be known for some time, but the movement toward employment has clearly accelerated and may not be easily reversible.

It also needs to be recognized that although the ACA has already undergone some changes and further modifications are likely, broad repeal and defunding of the entire legislation is not expected, given current majorities in Congress and the President's veto power. Suit has been filed in federal court by numerous organizations and a majority of states, challenging the constitutionality of the ACA, especially one central part relating to the individual mandate to obtain health insurance. At the time of writing, federal appellate judges are divided on the issue,[16] making it likely that these challenges will end up before the Supreme Court. Despite such legal and legislative challenges, the majority of the ACA will likely remain in place and the principles rooted in the law—that the uninsured should have health coverage and that clinicians and hospitals need to exhibit quality and efficiency value—will remain at the forefront of health care policy. Assuming that "this too shall pass" and that "things will look better in the morning"[17] would be a mistake. GI practitioners need to prepare, anticipate, and proactively "skate to where the puck will be."[18] The Administration's vision of the post-reform era has been clearly articulated by the Director of the White House Office of Health Reform, Nancy Min DeParle and her colleagues.[19]

These reforms will unleash forces that favor integration across the continuum of care. Some organizing function will need to be developed to track quality measures, account for and manage shared financial incentives, and oversee care coordination. Consequently, the health care system will evolve into one of two forms: organized around hospitals or organized around physician groups. ...Only hospitals or health plans can afford to make the necessary investments in information technology and management skills. This is not inevitable. As physicians organize themselves into increasingly larger groups- patient-centered medical home practices and accountable care organizations—they are, out of necessity, investing in information technology tools that are becoming both cheaper and more capable and investing in the acquisition or development of management skills that could provide these organizing functions efficiently for physician groups.[19]

THREE MAJOR TRENDS AND THEIR IMPACT ON THE INDEPENDENT GI PRACTICE
Demand for GI Services will Increase While Payments Continue to Decrease

Increased demand
The ACA increases access to health insurance coverage for United States citizens and legal residents by expanding Medicaid eligibility, by subsidizing private insurance premiums, and by cost sharing for certain lower-income individuals enrolled in health insurance exchanges. Starting in 2014, state Medicaid programs will be expanded to non-Medicare eligible individuals up to 133% of the federal poverty level (FPL), with subsidies for persons earning up to 400% of the FPL ($88,000 for a family of 4 in 2010), so their maximum "out-of-pocket" payment for annual premiums will be on a sliding scale from 2% to 9.8% of income.[20,21] State insurance exchanges will be created that provide access to private health insurance plans with standardized minimum benefit and cost-sharing packages for eligible individuals and small businesses. A tax penalty will be phased in for lack of coverage. The law prohibits denial of coverage and denial of claims based on pre-existing conditions. As a result of these changes, the number of insured

individuals is projected to increase by more than 32 million,[22] and half of these individuals will be covered by Medicaid (which traditionally pays an average of 72% of Medicare fees).[23] The ACA also eliminates copayments for Medicare and Medicaid enrollees for preventive screenings such as colorectal cancer screening examinations, and Medicare waives the deductible for such screenings. Private sector health plans are now required to provide a minimum benefits package and cover colorectal cancer and other preventive screenings, with no cost sharing for the patient.

Decreased payments
Many factors contribute to the continued decline in payments for GI services. Section 3134 of the ACA authorizes the Secretary of Health and Human Services (HHS) to adjust codes that are deemed "misvalued," with specific mention made of high-volume codes that have not been subject to review since the implementation of the current Resource Based Relative Value System. Several GI procedure codes fall into this category. The American Medical Association (AMA) Relative Value Update Committee has already begun an extensive review of these codes, and a downward adjustment of many GI code values and thus Medicare payments over the next few years is a likely outcome of this review. Much to the chagrin of physicians, the ACA does not address the Medicare physician payment update and the problematic Sustainable Growth Rate formula, thus leaving physicians at risk every year for additional significant cuts in Medicare reimbursement. Whether such cuts will continue to be avoided through Congressional action is anything but certain in times of increasing budget deficits. The sweep of new reimbursement models, yet to be developed, is also likely to include further efforts to redistribute income from specialists to primary care providers to address perceived payment inequalities.[24]

Among the most controversial provisions of the ACA is Section 3403, which establishes a 15-member Independent Payment Advisory Board (IPAB). Starting in 2015, the IPAB will make recommendations to Congress on lowering costs to the Medicare program. The recommendations will take effect unless Congress rejects the proposal and offers a recommendation that achieves the same savings. The board will be prohibited from making decisions that ration care, increase beneficiary premiums, or eliminate benefits, making health care providers the most likely parties to receive cuts. Opponents of the IPAB have raised concerns about possible rationing of care, and some lawmakers have expressed concern about ceding their jurisdiction to an unelected panel. Legislation and amendments to repeal the IPAB have been introduced, and could receive some attention during upcoming legislative discussions over deficit reduction and the fiscal budget for 2012.

The cumulative effect of these anticipated changes in demand and payments for GI services, together with the demographic trend of an aging population, is the imperative to care for more individuals at lower reimbursement levels. Practices will need to closely examine and understand their cost structure and profitability. Practices are well advised to conduct a "stress test" to determine whether they will still be economically viable if payments for GI services dropped by 20% to 30% and costs continue to increase at current rates. The pressure to gain efficiencies and drive down costs by eliminating waste will continue to intensify, favoring practice consolidation to be able to share resources and management capabilities. However, until the current fee-for-service system has been replaced with a new payment model, the opportunities for efficiency and revenue gains, and cost containment, will not change fundamentally. Optimizing endoscopy center and provider schedules and exploring additional revenue streams remains important. Practice models that rely on lower-cost nonphysician providers for office and inpatient work and maximize physician time in the endoscopy center will also help increase practice profitability. Although health care reform is not the only potentially transformative force, and disruptive technologies such as self-propelled endoscopes, remotely controlled capsules, and serum or stool DNA testing for colorectal cancer screening may eventually lead to a complete paradigm shift with regard to the demand of GI care, such changes do not appear to be imminent within the next few years.

Increased Emphasis on Quality, Value, and Transparency

The report by the Commonwealth Fund,[4] the Dartmouth Atlas project,[25] and many other studies, as well as commentaries in the lay press[26] have noted quality gaps and drawn public and political attention to the glaring variation in quality of care and resource use across the United States. As a result, there has been a growing interest in mandating that providers collect and report relevant quality and performance data, and improve the value of their care. Transparency of such quality measurement and improvement activities has been suggested as an important factor to enable patients to make informed choices about their care, enable purchasers to select higher-value health plans, and to motivate physicians to improve their performance.[27] In a recent study by the Commonwealth Fund,[28] 3 out of 4 health care opinion leaders considered increased transparency important for improving the health care system's performance.

The ACA mentions the word "value" 214 times and includes multiple related provisions. It increases incentive payments for physicians participating in Medicare's Physician Quality Reporting System (PQRS) through 2014. Starting in 2015, penalties will be assessed if providers do not successfully participate in the PQRS. The law also directs CMS to establish a hospital value-based purchasing program to pay hospitals based on performance on quality measures, and plans are to be developed to implement value-based purchasing programs for ambulatory surgical centers, home health agencies, and skilled nursing facilities. Furthermore, CMS is to develop a "value-based modifier," which will be applied to all physician payments starting in 2017.[29] The goal is to provide bonus payments to "high-value providers" while "low-value providers" will see their payments reduced. The details as to how CMS will reliably determine the quality and costs of individual providers remain to be determined. The CMS Physician Compare Web site[30] will be developed to make information on physician performance, including participation in PQRS, publicly available by 2013. The site can be expected to be similar to the Hospital Compare Web site already in operation.[31] Physicians should also be aware of private-sector initiatives such as the FAIR Health Web site launched in August of 2011.[32] This free online database now allows patients to look up the average charges for specific medical services in their area. The database arose out of two settlements with UnitedHealth Group (UHG) in 2009, when the AMA and state medical societies alleged that UHG used an intentionally flawed database to increase its profits by underpaying patients' medical bills. This new independent database could serve as a model for providing transparency and giving patients a better idea of what their financial responsibilities may be.

To remain successful in an era of transparency and practice and provider profiling, GI practices will have to proactively enter the "quality game." Practices have to understand and enter the national quality environment and establish a culture of quality improvement, with incentives to providers and staff around quality and performance measures. While many remain appropriately skeptical as to whether the quality of medical care can truly be measured in a meaningful fashion across all relevant clinical situations, payment and care decisions will be increasingly based on demonstrated value. Payors already have access to a large amount of performance data on providers, and stand ready to use that data for practice tiering by quality and cost. Health systems control an increasing percentage of primary care providers and will be able to build referral prompts into their electronic medical records that promote referrals to "high-performance" specialists. Practices should monitor local and national activities to identify evolving GI quality measure sets and begin implementing a basic set of measures that can be expanded and modified. Practices need to start telling their "quality story." Because patients perceive the quality of their experience more than they perceive the quality of their care, service excellence needs to be a key component of these performance improvement efforts, very much in line with the stated goal of the Triple Aim. The pursuit of clinical and service excellence will become increasingly broad, complex, and continuous, requiring a robust information technology (IT) infrastructure for data capture, aggregation, and analysis. The days of a "quality project" consisting of a manual review of a handful of paper charts are over. The GI practice that is able to demonstrate that it establishes, updates, and adheres to best practice guidelines, implements point-of-care decision tools, and benchmarks and distinguishes itself vis-a-vis competitors will do well in this new era of assessment and accountability, no matter what delivery and payment models will find widespread adoption.

Development of New Care Delivery and Payment Models

The ACA contains several provisions to create or study payment incentives and new service delivery models. Pilot projects such as those using bundled payments and shared savings contracts will encourage closer alignments between independent physician practices, hospitals, and payors. Collectively they represent a great shift of risk from the financiers of care to the providers of care.

Bundled payments

Effective 2013, the Secretary of HHS is instructed to establish pilot programs on payment bundling to encourage providers to improve care coordination to achieve savings for the Medicare program.[33] Bundled payment, also known as episode-based payment, may be defined as reimbursement "on the basis of expected costs for clinically defined episodes of care."[34,35] It has been described as a "middle ground"[36] between fee-for-service reimbursement and capitation (in which providers are paid a lump sum per patient regardless of how many services the patient receives). Considering the advantages and disadvantages of fee-for-service, pay for performance, bundled payment for episodes of care, and global payment such as capitation, Mechanic and Altman[37] concluded that "episode payments are the most immediately viable approach." Compared with fee-for-service, bundled payment is less likely to encourage unnecessary care and more likely to encourage coordination across providers, and potentially improves quality.[34] Moreover, because bundled payment approaches have been tested for years, real-life experience exists with this model. In 2007 the Geisinger Health System reported that a "ProvenCare" model for coronary artery bypass surgery that included best practices, patient engagement, and preoperative, inpatient, and postoperative care packaged into a fixed price led to shorter hospital stays and lower readmission rates in comparison with patients who received conventional care.[38] Researchers from the RAND Corporation estimated that national health care spending could be reduced by 5.4% between 2010 and 2019 if the PROMETHEUS model for bundled payment were widely used.[39]

Despite many open questions about bundled payments, addressed in numerous pilot projects by Medicare and various private payors, it seems likely, given the largely positive reports to date, that an increasing number of physician services will be paid via such bundling methodology in the future. GI practices need to prepare for this possibility by working to understand their average costs for discrete episodes of care as well as their cost range. Practices will need to implement a best-practice approach to defined care episodes, and need to benchmark themselves against other practices (and against themselves over time) to determine whether they can successfully offer "warranties" around specific care episodes for a bundled payment in a financially viable fashion. Their position in a competitive market will be enhanced by a lean cost structure, allowing the practice to derive a greater profit from the same episode-based payment. Practices with efficiently run AECs should be in a good position in this regard, relative to costlier, and often less efficient, hospital-based units.

Shared savings

While the new health care reform law encourages clinical integration in several pilot projects, perhaps the most direct encouragement is the Medicare Shared Savings Program for Accountable Care Organizations (ACOs). A more detailed discussion of ACOs by Komar appears elsewhere in this issue. In broad terms, they may be defined as networks of providers that can manage the full continuum of care for all patients within their network.[40] Should the ACO cut costs and achieve documented quality improvements, their providers are rewarded with a share of the savings. The expectation is that integration and care coordination will result in higher quality of care and lower costs.[5,40] Perhaps no part of the ACA has generated more activity on the part of provider organizations. Hospitals and physician groups are exploring ways to align and connect now to be ready for the future,[41] and provider groups are spending considerable efforts and money to make sure they make the transition correctly. As an example, about 80 provider organizations are studying ACOs in the Accountable Care Organization Learning Network, a joint project of the Engelberg Center for Health Care Reform at the Brookings Institution and the Dartmouth Institute for Health Policy and Clinical Practice. The program offers members monthly webinars and an ability to share best practices.[42] Meanwhile, commercial insurers who fear losing business to ACOs, and who may want to take on the financial risk of contracting directly with employers and patients, are building their own ACOs. United-Health Group, through its Optum Health subsidiary, is making significant investments (rumored to be in the $1 billion range) to position itself as a leader of the emerging ACO field by buying medical groups and launching physician management groups throughout the country.[43] Humana and WellPoint are said to be pursuing a similar strategy.[44]

There are many challenges associated with implementing ACOs,[45] and it will be several years before the results from various pilot projects can provide some insight as to what a successful ACO might look like and whether the predominant model will be structured as an integrated health system, a large multispecialty group, an independent practice association, a payer-owned organization, or an entirely different concept yet to be developed. GI practices need to become familiar with the various ACO models, explore the evolving dynamics in their local markets, and monitor this issue very closely, as it may truly revolutionize the way medical care is being provided in the future as well as the role independent practices can play in the provision of such care.

TRANSFORMATION OF THE INDEPENDENT GI PRACTICE MODEL

What do the ACA provisions and the related trends mean for independent GI practices? The increase in demand for GI services and the imperative to provide higher-quality care, at less cost, through novel delivery and payment models with greater transparency and better care coordination between providers will require investments that will be difficult to afford for independent physicians, especially those in smaller practices. Practice transformation and consolidation will be inevitable in most markets.

A solid IT infrastructure with a well-integrated electronic health record (EHR) and the ability to track clinical and operational performance measures is indispensable. If practices have not yet adopted an EHR, they will have to do so; if they are using an ineffective disjointed EHR, they may have to change to a more functional system. While hospitals are now commonly encouraging local practices to adopt their hospital electronic medical record, GI practices need to carefully consider the desired local alignments but also the necessary core functionalities needed to support GI services. As an ambulatory, procedure-oriented specialty, a well-interfaced endoscopy writer and office EHR with build-in best practices and point-of-care decision support tools for GI services should be the backbone of any GI practice IT infrastructure. An integrated practice management module with good data analytics, and a patient portal to support the increasing trend toward electronic/telemedicine will also be necessary. External interfaces with the major hospital EHRs in the region will promote care coordination. To date, EHRs have a mixed record as a means of saving labor and extending the physician workforce. Installing an EHR requires a considerable amount of physician time and often results in lost productivity. Under the Health Information Technology for Economic and Clinical Health Act of 2009 (HITECH), providers that implement a certified EHR and comply with Meaningful Use guidelines are eligible to receive incentives of up to $44,000,[46,47] but this is not likely to cover all costs associated with such an implementation. A study by the Physicians Foundation notes that it costs a minimum of $35,000 per physician to implement an EHR, and $15,000 annually per physician to maintain an EHR, not factoring in lost productivity while systems are being installed.[48] Nevertheless, the redesign of patient care, the need to improve efficiency, safety, and quality of care, and the collaboration required among providers will make EHRs a mandatory component for most if not all practices.

Hospital Employment and Other Evolving Practice Models

As a result the forces described, an increasing number of gastroenterologists are giving up independent practice in favor of hospital employment. Even prior to the current health reform efforts, there has been a steady decline of private medical practice in the United States at an annual rate of about 2% per year for the past 25 years.[49] While the greater part of this decline initially occurred in primary care and was largely driven by low reimbursement for primary care services, the number of independent specialty practices is now also decreasing at a significant pace. The reasons for this shift are complex and include generational, demographic, and financial issues, and the ACA is accelerating this trend. Hospitals, in turn, are motivated to buy up physician groups and solo practitioners in an effort to create the kind of coordinated medical teams that federal health care reform puts a premium on,[50] and to increase their leverage with an also rapidly consolidating payor world. According to a recent survey by the Medical Group Management Association, 2008 marked the first year when more physicians were employed by hospitals than were in independent practice.[51] While becoming part of a large integrated health system allows access to clinical, financial, and managerial resources, it comes at the significant price of relinquishing autonomy and ultimate strategic decision-making authority to health system administrators. It may turn out to be the correct position if the health system evolves as a dominant player and moves aggressively to control all medical care in a market. One may surmise that care coordination and overall efficiencies will be improved if all physicians work under one roof, but data to back up this assumption are actually scarce. There is some concern that the ability to make important purchasing and other strategic decisions to optimize operations for a high-throughput, technology-driven and mostly ambulatory specialty such as GI may be compromised by competing health system priorities, with the potential for negative effects on patient care. The effects on the cost of care for GI services are also far from certain. Anecdotally some practices that have sold their AECs to health systems have seen these centers being converted to hospital-based endoscopy units, which are now providing the same endoscopic services at increased costs to patients and the health care system at large. Some general concerns about provider integration with large health systems also apply to GI. As an example, how the physician-patient relationship will be changed when providers are "at-will employees," and whether they will be able to advocate for patient interests in the same way they do as independent providers, remains to be seen.

Whether a GI practice will be forced to sell to the local health system or have access to other potential practice models will be largely determined by its specific local environment and the position it has been able to attain in that market. For some, joining forces in a larger single-specialty GI practice or a multispecialty group may be an alternative option. Entirely new arrangements may also evolve, such as the formation of a national single-specialty practice consortium that may be able to bring GI practices together around a common IT platform to jointly pursue best clinical practices, performance measurement and enhancement, and a multitude of purchasing and revenue cycle management activities.

In addition to the need for capital and management resources to affect the necessary practice transformation, the access to primary care referral streams for endoscopic procedures is a key consideration. Depending on the local circumstances and the practice's ability to promote itself as the high-value (high quality, low cost) provider of GI care in its region, it may well be feasible, even mutually beneficial, for some practices to remain organizationally independent but strategically aligned with local health systems and other accountable care organizations to jointly provide well-coordinated care. Health systems are finding themselves under great pressure to reduce costs, and it may well be too costly for them to own all specialists for the long term.[9] Hospital CEOs acknowledge that some of their best relationships with physicians are with nonemployed providers and that such relationships can lead to creative and innovative strategies to deliver health care while benefiting both the hospital system and privately owned practice.

In conclusion, it seems likely that the GI practice model in the postreform era will not be a "one size fits all" model. Models such as practice consolidation with the formation of larger single-specialty GI practices or multispecialty groups, hospital employment, ACOs, and others will vary by region and market. The small "low-tech" practice model will be largely replaced. Integration across the continuum of care will be necessary to achieve care coordination. However, whether such integration has to equate to full employment or if effective strategic alignments between different providers and systems are possible while maintaining operational independence remains to be seen. As we enter this great experiment of United States health care reform, it is worth remembering that the optimal delivery model has yet to be developed and validated. Which practice model will ultimately prevail and become the dominant model of medical care in the United States depends not to an insignificant degree on the outcome of the health care reform implementation efforts over the next decade.

REFERENCES

1. Organization for Economic Development. OECD Health Data 2011, published June 2011. Available at: www.oecd.org/health/healthdata. Accessed August 25, 2011.
2. Sisko AM, Truffer CJ, Keehan SP, et al. National health spending projections: the estimated impact of reform through 2019. Health Aff (Millwood) 2010;29(10):1933–41.
3. Littenberg G. Where will health reform take GI practice? Gastrointest Endosc 2010;72(2):396–400.
4. Davis K, Schoen C, Schoenbaum SC, et al. Mirror, mirror on the wall: an international update on the comparative performance of American health care. New York: The Commonwealth Fund; 2007. Available at: http://www.commonwealthfund.org/Publications/Fund-Reports/2007/May/Mirror–Mirror-on-the-Wall–An-International-Update-on-the-Comparative-Performance-of-American-Healt.aspx. Accessed August 25, 2011.
5. Dorn SD. United States health care reform in 2009. A primer for gastroenterologists. Clin Gastroenterol Hepatol 2009;7:1168–73.
6. Berwick DM, Nolan TW, Whittington J. The triple aim: care, health, and cost. Health Aff (Millwood) 2008;27(3):759–69.
7. Gawande A. Cowboys and pit crews. Harvard Medical School Commencement Address, 2011. Available at: http://www.hcfms.com/Uploads/SharedDocuments/GawandeCommencement2011.pdf. Accessed August 25, 2011.
8. Frakes JT. Outpatient endoscopy. The case for the ambulatory surgery center. Gastrointest Endosc Clin N Am 2002;12(2):215–27.
9. Vicari JJ. The future value of ambulatory endoscopy centers in the United States. Challenges and opportunities. Gastrointest Endosc, in press.
10. Available at: http://www.gpo.gov/fdsys/pkg/PLAW-111publ148/content-detail.html. Accessed August 31, 2011.
11. Available at: http://www.gpo.gov/fdsys/pkg/PLAW-111publ152/content-detail.html. Accessed August 31, 2011.
12. Available at: http://www.recovery.gov/About/Pages/The_Act.aspx. Accessed August 31, 2011.
13. Available at: http://www.kff.org/healthreform/upload/8061.pdf. Accessed August 31, 2012.
14. Available at: http://www.loc.gov/crsinfo. Accessed August 31, 2011.
15. Available at: http://www.ama-assn.org/ama1/pub/upload/mm/399/hr3590-summary-of-provisions.pdf. Accessed August 31, 2011.
16. Available at: http://online.wsj.com/article/SB10001424053111904006104576504383685080762.html. Accessed August 28, 2011.
17. Bagheera to Mowgli in "The Jungle Book" (Walt Disney's 1967 animated film version of Rudyard Kipling's story).
18. Wayne Gretzky. Available at: http://en.wikipedia.org/wiki/Wayne_Gretzky. Accessed September 28, 2011.
19. Kocher R, Emanuel EJ, DeParle NA. The Affordable Care Act and the future of clinical medicine: the opportunities and challenges. Ann Intern Med 2010;153:536–9.
20. Holahan J, Dom S. What is the impact of the Patient Protection and Affordable Care Act (PPACA) on the States? Available at: http://www.rwjf.org/files/research/65049.pdf. Accessed August 31, 2011.
21. Foster RS. Estimated financial effects of the "Patient Protection and Affordable Care Act," as amended. memorandum. Baltimore (MD): Centers for Medicare and Medicaid Services; 2010. Available at: http://www.cms.gov/ActuarialStudies/Downloads/PPACA_2010-04-22.pdf. Accessed August 31, 2011.

22. Kaiser Family Foundation. The uninsured: a primer. Key facts about Americans without health insurance. Available at: http://www.kff.org/uninsured/upload/7451-06.pdf. Accessed August 31, 2011.
23. Medicaid-to-Medicare fee index. Available at: http://www.statehealthfacts.org/comparetable.jsp?ind=196&cat=4. Accessed August 31, 2011.
24. Vladeck BC. Fixing Medicare's physician payment system. N Engl J Med 2010; 362:1955–7.
25. Available at: http://www.dartmouthatlas.org. Accessed August 31, 2011.
26. Gawande A. The cost conundrum. Available at: http://www.newyorker.com/reporting/2009/06/01/090601fa_fact_gawande. Accessed August 31, 2010.
27. Colmers JM. Commonwealth Fund Commission on a high performance health system. Public reporting and transparency. New York: The Commonwealth Fund; 2007.
28. Shea KK, Shih A, Davis K. Commonwealth Fund Commission on a high performance health system data brief: health care opinion leaders' views on health care delivery system reform. New York: The Commonwealth Fund; 2008.
29. Ginsburg PB. Rapidly evolving physician-payment policy-more than the SGR. N Engl J Med 2011;364:172–6.
30. Available at: http://www.medicare.gov/find-a-doctor/provider-search.aspx. Accessed August 31, 2011.
31. Available at: http://www.hospitalcompare.hhs.gov. Accessed August 31, 2011.
32. Available at: http://fairhealthconsumer.org. Accessed August 31, 2011.
33. Bundled payments—Medicare pilot program. Health reform GPS: a joint project of the George Washington University and the Robert Wood Johnson Foundation. Available at: http://healthreformgps.org/resources/bundled-payments-%E2%80%93-medicare-pilot-program. Accessed August 31, 2011.
34. Miller HD. From volume to value: better ways to pay for health care. Health Aff (Millwood) 2009;28(5):1418–28.
35. Satin DJ, Miles J. Performance based bundled payments: potential benefits and burdens. Minn Med 2009;92(10):33–5.
36. RAND Corporation. Overview of bundled payment. Available at: http://www.randcompare.org/policy-options/bundled-payment. Accessed August 31, 2011.
37. Mechanic RE, Altman SH. Payment reform options: episode payment is a good place to start. Health Aff (Millwood) 2009;28(2):262–71.
38. Casale AS, Paulus RA, Selna MJ, et al. "ProvenCare": a provider-driven pay-for-performance program for acute episodic cardiac surgical care. Ann Surg 2007; 246(4):613–21.
39. Hussey PS, Eibner C, Ridgely MS, et al. Controlling U.S. health care spending—separating promising from unpromising approaches. N Engl J Med 2009;361(22): 2109–11.
40. Fisher ES, McClellan MB, Bertko J, et al. Fostering accountable health care: moving forward in Medicare. Health Aff (Millwood) 2009;28(2):219–31.
41. Levey, N. Healthcare law has more doctors teaming up. Los Angeles Times. July 28, 2010. Available at: http://articles.latimes.com/2010/jul/28/nation/la-na-health-doctors-20100728. Accessed September 28, 2011.
42. The Brookings Institution. Overview of the 2009-2010 Brookings-Dartmouth ACO Learning Network. 2010. Available at: https://xteam.brookings.edu/bdacoln/Pages/OverviewoftheNetworkMembership.aspx. Accessed August 31, 2010.
43. WSJ: United buying doctors. Available at: http://online.wsj.com/article/SB10001424053111903895904576542553422509280.html. Accessed August 31, 2011.

44. Weaver C. Managed care enters the exam room as insurers buy doctor groups. Available at: www.kaiserhealthnews.org/Stories/2011/July/01/unitedhealth-insurers-buy-doctors-groups.aspx. Accessed August 25, 2011.
45. Singer S, Shortell SM. Implementing accountable care organizations. Ten potential mistakes and how to learn from them. JAMA 2011;306(7):758–9.
46. Blumenthal D, Tavenner M. The "meaningful use" regulation for electronic health records. N Engl J Med 2010;363(6):501–4.
47. Brill JV, Kosinski LR. What GI practices need to know about meaningful EHR use. 2011. Available at: http://www.gastro.org/aga_meaningful_use.pdf. Accessed August 25, 2011.
48. Available at: http://www.physiciansfoundation.org/uploadedFiles/PF_Survey_Report_Nov08.pdf. Accessed August 31, 2011.
49. Isaacs SL, Jellinek PS, Ray WL. The independent physician—going, going. N Engl J Med 2009;360(7):655–8.
50. Kocher R, Sahni NR. Hospitals race to employ physicians—the logic behind a money-losing proposition. N Engl J Med 2011;364:1790–3.
51. Cantlupe J. Physician alignment in an era of change. Brentwood (TN): HealthLeaders Media; 2010. Available at: http://www.healthleadersmedia.com/page-2/MAG-256427/Physician-Alignment-in-an-Era-of-Change. Accessed August 31, 2011.

Impact of Health Care Reform on Academic Medical Centers

Ian L. Taylor, MD, PhD, AGAF*, Ross McVicker Clinchy, PhD

KEYWORDS

• Health care reform • Academic medical centers
• Accountable care organizations

The Patient Protection and Affordable Care Act (PPACA) was signed into United States law[1] by President Barack Obama on March 23, 2010 and was followed swiftly by the Healthcare and Education Reconciliation Act (HECA) of 2010,[2] which contained significant modifications to the PPACA. The legislation has defined broad goals for health care reform including the provision of high-quality, affordable health care for all Americans.[3] The Congressional Budget Office[4] has estimated that it will provide coverage to more than 95% of all Americans while reducing the federal deficit by $138 billion over the next 10 years with additional reductions in the following years. These two goals—expanding coverage while reducing costs—may, at least on the surface, appear to be contradictory, and the methods intended to achieve them may seem overly complex and the actual results hard to predict. In general, however, it seems that even if the impact of these changes was evenly distributed across the entire system, some sectors, including those most closely linked to academic medicine, will experience seismic changes. Moreover, the authors suggest that the changes may not be evenly distributed but will instead disproportionately affect academic medical centers (AMCs).

The PPACA will affect all of the nation's AMCs, as well as the health care provider system in general, but its impact will be most profound on those centers that have incorporated one or more safety-net hospitals in their system. The law has been subject to legal challenges regarding its constitutionality in various lower-level federal courts, which have come down on both sides of the argument,[5] and a final decision will be made by the Supreme Court, which will likely hear arguments in 2012. For the purposes of these discussions, however, it is assumed that the laws will remain largely intact. The provisions within the PPACA and HECA that may disproportionately affect AMCs are discussed in this article.

The authors have nothing to disclose.
SUNY Downstate Medical Center, Dean's Office, School of Medicine, 450 Clarkson Avenue, Box 97, Brooklyn, NY 11203, USA
* Corresponding author.
E-mail address: Ian.Taylor@downstate.edu

Gastrointest Endoscopy Clin N Am 22 (2012) 29–37
doi:10.1016/j.giec.2011.08.005
1052-5157/12/$ – see front matter © 2012 Elsevier Inc. All rights reserved.

giendo.theclinics.com

EXPANDED ELIGIBILITY FOR MEDICAID

One approach to the expansion of coverage is the provision that would make all nonelderly Americans with incomes below 133% of the Federal Poverty Level eligible for Medicaid,[1,2] and it has been estimated that under the PPACA 16 million additional Americans will be covered by Medicaid. Spending per Medicaid enrollee varies widely from region to region, but $5000 per enrollee per year is a reasonable (and conservative) basis for a "back of the envelope" calculation, yielding an annual expenditure of $80 billion for this new population—an expenditure that is, in many states, shared by the state and federal governments. This increased expense, whatever it turns out to be, is to be (more than) balanced by reductions in other areas.[6]

REDUCTIONS IN DISPROPORTIONATE SHARE HOSPITAL PAYMENT

One such source is the Disproportionate Share Hospital (DSH) payments by Medicare and Medicaid, which are to be reduced[1,2] and phased out to help cover the costs of covering more people under Medicaid. DSH payments have in the past supplemented the direct payments by Medicaid and Medicare to hospitals, to compensate them for the costs of caring for the uninsured and the indigent and, therefore, are especially critical to the public and other "safety-net" hospitals that care for many of these patients.

Under the new legislation, Medicare and Medicaid Designated Health Services cuts and other Centers for Medicare and Medicaid Services (CMS) reductions beginning in 2010 will amount to a $158 billion reduction over 10 years. Medicare update factors to hospitals will be reduced by $112 billion beginning in 2010. Medicare DSH will be reduced $22 billion starting in 2010 and Medicaid DSH will be reduced $14 billion beginning in 2014. In theory, the expansion of coverage to include many of the currently uninsured who seek care at AMCs would help offset the loss of DSH payments. Unfortunately, that will not be the case for hospitals in AMCs that currently serve as safety nets for the uninsured.

There are several reasons for this. In most venues, the current Medicaid payments do not fully cover the cost of care, suggesting that an increase in the numbers covered by Medicaid will constitute an additional financial burden that will become even more problematic when coupled with the loss of DSH payments that previously helped cover the cost of care for the uninsured. The Massachusetts experience, in which a sweeping health care reform that bears a striking resemblance to the PPACA was enacted,[7–9] reduced DSH payments to hospitals to help offset the costs of increased health care coverage paid by the government. A recent article,[8] however, indicated that the reductions in DSH and other payments by the state had been devastating to Boston Medical Center and the safety-net hospitals in Massachusetts. Indeed, Boston Medical Center has sued the state of Massachusetts, claiming it was covering too much of the cost for expanded medical coverage.

Another concern is the future trajectory of the Medicaid rates. Although the Massachusetts health care reform was slated to increase Medicaid payment rates to hospitals from 80% to 95% of costs, the Massachusetts Hospital Association indicated the real rate of Medicaid reimbursement had fallen to 75% of actual costs.[7] In the past, hospitals had managed to cross-subsidize with excess funds from patients covered by private insurance.[10] However, this will become increasingly more difficult, if not impossible, as health care reform is rolled out over the next 10 years.[11]

IMPACT OF THE PPACA ON FACULTY PRACTICE PLANS

Although safety-net hospitals in AMCs have been significantly aided in the past by the DSH payments, fee-for-service Medicaid has never been a good payer for physician professional services.[12] (In 2008, Medicaid physician fee payments in the United States were >75% of the Medicare fee schedule.) As a result, many physicians feel forced to decline new Medicaid patients, and there does not appear to be any provision within the PPACA to change that situation to any significant degree. The PPACA does contain a requirement that the Medicaid payment rates to primary care physicians be no less than 100% of Medicare payment rates in 2013 and 2014, but this increased rate will only be available to primary care physicians for those 2 years.[1,2] These increased rates will not apply to subspecialty professional services. As a result, referral of the increased population of Medicaid patients to subspecialists will be problematic[12] as payments to specialists will continue to be insufficient to cover costs. AMCs, for better or worse, have been oriented around the provision of subspecialty care, and shifting to a primary care–based, gatekeeper system will present a cultural and financial challenge. It is anticipated that many more physicians not employed by hospitals will opt out of Medicaid.[12] Although physicians currently have the option to opt out of Medicaid, hospitals do not. Patients will be forced to seek care for urgent and emergent care at hospital emergency rooms (ERs) if the problem of access is not addressed.[8,9] This increased burden will likely fall on AMCs to a disproportionate degree, and these centers will be ill equipped to accommodate this need if they maintain their subspecialty focus.

The Association of American Medical Colleges (AAMC)[7] noted that 36.9% of patients covered by "public insurance" after health care reform in Massachusetts had difficulty obtaining care in the prior 12 months compared with only 16.9% of Medicare beneficiaries. This finding was in part due to fewer physician offices accepting patients covered by Medicaid. In 2005, 79% of Internal Medicine groups in Massachusetts accepted Medicaid patients. This figure dropped to 60% in 2009. These figures may explain the observation that total ER visits have increased significantly in Massachusetts since the introduction of health care reform, despite predictions that the use of the ERs would decrease. Medicaid patients had the highest proportion (55%) of their ER visits considered preventable or avoidable. It is worth noting that when Massachusetts introduced health care reform, it had more physicians than any other state in the union and a low uninsured population compared with the rest of country. As such, AMCs in other regions of the country are likely to see greater problems relative to access and increased waiting time to see physicians for all patients once the PPACA is fully introduced.

UNDOCUMENTED IMMIGRANTS AND THE REMAINING UNINSURED

Undocumented immigrants and migrant workers, whose numbers are thought to exceed 12 million, will not be eligible for health care insurance under the PPACA.[1,2] These individuals and their families will still need health care, and are likely to continue to seek that care at safety-net hospitals within AMCs. The costs of this care will largely be borne by the hospitals and their parent AMCs, as these costs will not be reimbursed.

In addition, the Massachusetts experience suggests that despite the development of Health Insurance Exchanges and the threat of financial penalties, the PPACA underestimates the numbers of Americans who will continue without private health care insurance.[10] These patients will also seek emergent medical care at safety-net hospitals, the cost of which will also not be reimbursed. The question arises as to whether hospital administrators and health care workers will be forced into the role of "PPACA police," charged with reporting individuals who refuse to pay for health insurance or who are in the country illegally.

Many other ethical issues will arise in terms of the delivery of care to illegal immigrants and the uninsured who require urgent or emergent care. It is estimated that 23 million people will fall into these two categories. However, this figure is likely an underestimate.[10]

IMPLICATIONS FOR GRADUATE AND UNDERGRADUATE MEDICAL EDUCATION

Historically, the teaching hospitals that train residents have been reimbursed for the increased costs this entails both through Direct Medical Education (DME) and Indirect Medical Education (IME) payments. These payments vary widely across different regions, and IME payments usually exceed the DME payments that cover resident salaries.

Federal support of resident training has not changed since 1997 when Congress limited the number of training slots supported by CMS as part of the Balanced Budget Act, and the PPACA does not do enough to change this. Instead, the PPACA[1,2] will require CMS to take 65% of the DME and IME supported residency slots that have gone unused and redistribute them according to specified criteria. The remaining 35% will no longer be supported by CMS. The health care reform bill requires that CMS allocate 70% of the redistributed slots to hospitals in states with resident-to-population ratios in the lowest quartile, and 30% of the slots to hospitals located either in the 10 states with the highest proportion of their population living in a health professional shortage area or in rural areas. The impact of this redistribution on AMCs will vary significantly on a regional basis. Moreover, the future of both DME and IME payments is uncertain, as Congress is currently discussing draconian cuts to graduate medical education as part of its deficit reduction plans.

The PPACA also fails to address the inadequate number of total residency slots available, given the predictions of significant physician shortages.[13] The AAMC[13] estimates that the United States will have 91,500 too few physicians by 2020 and that the shortage will grow to 130,000 in 2025. Physician shortages are anticipated in both primary care and in the subspecialties, and are based in part on the growth and aging of the United States population. The other major driving force will be health care reform itself, which could lead to 32 million newly covered Americans seeking health care, and health care use is anticipated to be higher in this group than for those with current insurance coverage.[12,14] Kathleen Sebelius, Health and Human Services (HHS) Secretary, estimates[15] only 16,000 additional primary care providers will result from the stimulus monies that the government will allocate in the next 5 years.

Finally, based on the AAMC's predictions of a physician shortage, United States medical schools were encouraged to expand their medical school class size, and approximately 20 new allopathic medical schools were started. Schools of Osteopathy have increased at an even greater rate and offshore schools have expanded at an astonishing rate. Although the AAMC estimates that United States medical school enrollment will soon have expanded by about one third, there has been no commensurate increase in the number of residencies available for graduate training. This trend will make competition for the available training positions even more intense than it currently is. Unless this problem is addressed, there will be insufficient physicians to address all the health care needs of the large number of newly insured Americans.

THE PPACA AND THE HEALTH CARE DELIVERY SYSTEM

The new legislation[1,2] does, however, attempt to stimulate innovation directed toward the reform of the delivery system in order to absorb the impact of the expansion of coverage and shifts in funding.

Health Information Technology

The PPACA[1,2] contains a provision for hospitals to receive federal incentive payments for "meaningful use" of Health Information Technology. Hospitals are embracing electronic medical records systems and e-prescribing.[16] Hospitals are also experimenting with e-consults and telemedicine to improve efficiency in anticipation of the millions of newly insured patients who will enter the health care system. The costs of these technologic transitions are substantial, and it seems likely that many AMCs with safety-net hospitals under stress from the developments already described will not be able to afford them,[14] thus placing them at a disadvantage as they compete to receive government funding based on "meaningful use" of health information technology. An amount of $26 billion has been allocated in the Recovery Act[14] to stimulate adoption of health care information technology that will bring added benefits. New avenues of clinical research will be built around the electronic medical record, given the ready accessibility of clinical outcomes data, which will lead to additional funding opportunities. Such data will also aid standardization of care that will save costs while improving quality.

New Systems of Health Care Delivery

If the analysis to this point is correct, the huge influx of Americans newly covered by Medicaid will not be able to access the health care system through the private sector. Without a fundamental redesign of this nation's health care system, the PPACA is destined to fail. The PPACA[1,2] directs a new Center for Medicare and Medicaid Innovation to evaluate and test new care delivery models including Healthcare Innovation Zones (HIZs), which the PPACA defines as "groups of providers that include a teaching hospital, physicians and other clinical entities that, through their structure, operations and joint activity, deliver a full spectrum of integrated and comprehensive health care services to applicable individuals while also incorporating methods for the clinical training of future health care professionals." Health care delivery by HIZs must become more cost effective and provide high-quality, patient-focused care. It is in the design and implementation of new systems of care that AMCs can and should find a unique place in health care reform. However, the great fear for AMCs is that the safety-net hospitals with which they are associated, and which constitute a major focus of graduate and undergraduate teaching, will continue to be the focus of care for the uninsured and underinsured in the new health care system without the funds that had previously supported them in the past. As a result, the safety-net hospitals that the uninsured have depended upon in emergency situations may no longer be in existence, given the massive decreases in Medicare and Medicaid payments to these institutions. This situation will in turn radically change the environment in which health care professionals are educated and trained.

Section 3022 of the PPACA[1] establishes the Medicare Shared Saving Program (MSSP) for Accountable Care Organizations (ACOs), which is one approach that AMCs will undoubtedly explore. The goal of MSSP is to achieve better care for individuals, better health for populations, and slower growth in costs through improvements in care. An ACO must assume responsibility for the care of a clearly defined population of Medicare beneficiaries and, if it succeeds in delivering high-quality care while reducing costs, it will share in the cost savings with Medicare. However, the ACO will receive less monies than it would have under the old fee-for-service reimbursement and, even if the ACO saved 10% of the prior year's cost of caring for this defined population, it would receive only a portion of the savings (eg, 50% of the 10% saved) as a bonus at the end of the year.

As such, the major challenge for AMCs is that an ACO must assume a degree of financial risk as they move from fee-for-service to bundled payments,[16] without a high level of certainty that they will be successful or that the financial returns for success will justify the investments required. Such ventures into uncharted territory with uncertain results will be daunting for institutions that are already struggling to cope with the impact of the reforms described here. This scenario suggests that the institutions with the greatest intellectual capital may also be the ones that lack financial capital, which may effectively bar them from participation in what is clearly an important effort for our society and our economy.

Moreover, ACOs taking part in the MSSP will probably also be required to develop a strong foundation of primary care—something that may be both difficult and expensive, given that AMCs have been built in the past on subspecialty care.[16,17] In addition, AMCs, which have been risk averse in the past,[16] will have to accept some risk here, knowing that prior attempts to build comprehensive care networks by purchasing primary care practices have historically proved to be costly mistakes for many AMCs. However, in the past this approach was built on the concept of buying a sufficiently large referral network to support the AMC's subspecialists. This concept proved to be flawed. Under the ACO paradigm, the primary care physician is the gatekeeper and health care manager who becomes key to controlling the cost in a system in which reimbursement shifts from fee-for-service to bundled payments. This approach is reflected in HHS Secretary Kathleen Sebelius' statement[15] that "I believe the new accountable care organization model will help us eliminate redundant services that drive up costs."

The reforms will force AMCs to decide whether becoming an ACO is a financially viable option for them. The cultural barriers inherent within AMCs that will have to be overcome if the AMC is to provide high-quality, patient-focused care while assuming financial risk are substantial.[18] On the positive side, Griner[11] has argued that a shift to bundled payments from our current fee-for-service system "is more consistent with AMCs' core values" and that adoption of these new health care delivery systems will benefit the AMCs' teaching and service missions through a renewed focus on the quality of care and a more discriminating use of health care resources. In his view, this will lead to a better educational environment for students and residents that stresses bedside skills and avoids unnecessary tests.

Berkowitz and Miller[19] also see health care reform as an opportunity for AMCs "to modernize their approaches to research, education and care." These investigators believe that AMCs are "well positioned to spearhead efforts to develop, pilot and disseminate new patient-focused measures and models of care." Berkowitz and Miller[19] point to new sources of funding that the PPACA brings within the Patient-Centered Outcomes Research Institute ($500 million in research funding annually by 2015) and the Center for Medicare and Medicaid Innovation with $10 billion to spend over 10 years to support innovation grants and to develop new care delivery models. However, they also stress that each AMC will have to assess whether it is positioned to assume the financial risk associated with becoming an ACO, emphasizing that AMCs will have to abandon departmentally based care in favor of multidisciplinary centers to promote patient-centered care. In addition, Berkowitz and Miller[19] believe that AMCs' promotion and tenure system will need to change so that it appropriately recognizes faculty's contributions to high-quality, cost-effective patient care.

POTENTIAL IMPACT OF ACOs ON SUBSPECIALISTS IN AMCs

The regulations proposed by the CMS for ACOs are focused primarily on enhanced access to primary care providers rather than to specialists, including gastroenterologists. The lack of attention to subspecialty care reflects an assumption that such care is less cost effective and that all care must be shifted through the primary care sector. However, for patients with complex, chronic diseases, quality care often involves a team approach in which a specialist may be the more appropriate care coordinator. Subspecialists may be in the best position to provide the best quality and cost-effective care for complex diseases. CMS' ACO model creates a primary care gatekeeper model that, in other settings, has created barriers to appropriate care by incorporating financial disincentives to referral to the appropriate subspecialist. Furthermore, many specialists already function as the primary care provider to Medicare patients with chronic diseases. At the very least CMS needs to develop explicit guidelines for how referrals to specialists are to occur, to ensure appropriate transitions of care under the PPACA. It is likely that some AMCs may remain subspecialty focused and subcontract with other ACOs for care of patients with complex chronic diseases.

The PPACA[1] makes the measurement of quality of care an integral component of an ACO program. This component includes accountability for the overall health of a defined patient population that is built on a coordinated delivery of health care services. The PPACA[1] also encourages investment in IT infrastructure and the redesign of care processes to deliver high-quality and efficient service delivery. The CMS has identified 65 measures on which ACOs will report to allow an assessment of the quality of care being delivered.[17] However, very few relate to specialist care and only one to gastroenterologists (colon cancer screening rates). Lack of meaningful quality measures for specialists largely excludes them from meaningful involvement in the financial incentives to ACOs to improve quality. This fact will affect most AMCs given their specialty-based structure.

The American Hospital Association[20] estimates that it would cost between $11.6 million and $26.1 million to build the ACO infrastructure and run it for the first year. By contrast, the CMS estimated these costs to be only $1.8 million.[20] CMS' ACO proposal is based on evidence the agency collected during the Physician Group Practice (PGP) demonstration.[17,21] The participating organizations were predominantly large AMCs with well-established infrastructures. Despite this, only half of the participants in the PGP demonstration were able to share in the financial incentives under the Shared Savings Program. Furthermore, none of the participants managed to recoup their initial investment by the third year. CMS' ACO appears to transfer too much risk to the new organization relative to the potential rewards, and it may need to consider providing capital to fund the infrastructure required to establish physician-led or hospital-led ACOs.

SUMMARY

The authors, like most Americans, support both of the primary goals of health care reform: the expansion of coverage to "near-universal" levels and the containment of the cost of health care to a level that our economy can sustain. Taken together, these goals can be integrated into the challenge of how to provide good-quality health care for all of the roughly 300 million Americans—children, adult women and men, the elderly, and disabled—perhaps at an average cost of something like $10,000 per person per year, or $3 trillion a year in expenditure. (The most recent projections for 2020 are for a total cost of over $4 trillion and an average cost of $13,000 per

American.) This is not to say that academic medicine can come up with all the answers alone, and one must be well aware of the characteristics that will make it difficult for academic medicine to take up this challenge, or that critics may see academic medicine as a significant "part of the problem." The authors also believe, however, that the deep expertise in the diagnosis and treatment of disease, the expertise in working collaboratively with teams of health care professionals, the perspective that a culture of investigation can bring to the questions of comparative effectiveness that academic medicine can bring to bear on these problems—and the fact that most of the next generation of doctors, nurses, and other allied health professionals are being, and will be, trained in these venues—means that AMCs can and must be part of the solution.

REFERENCES

1. Patient Protection and Affordable Care Act. Public Law 111-148. Enacted March 23, 2010.
2. The Healthcare and Education Reconciliation Act. Public Law enacted March 30, 2010.
3. The Obama plan: stability and security for all Americans. Available at: www.whitehouse.gov. Accessed June 7, 2011.
4. Congressional budget office, cost estimates for HR 4872, reconciliation act of 2010. Available at: http://www.cbo.gov/doc.cfm?index=11379&type=1. Accessed June 7, 2011.
5. Hall AM. Healthcare reform—what went wrong on the way to the courthouse. N Engl J Med 2011;364(4):295-7.
6. Sommers BD, Epstein AM. Medicaid expansion—the soft underbelly of health care reform? N Engl J Med 2010;362(22):2085-7.
7. Schulman SA. Preparing for United States health care reform: what we can learn from Massachusetts. Association of American Medical Colleges, Center for Workforce Studies; 2011. Available at: http://www.AAMC.org. Accessed July 21, 2011.
8. Beaty P. Will safety net hospital survive health reform? Available at: http://www.msnbc.msn.com/cleanprint/CleanPrintProxy.aspx?unique=1311277308444. Accessed July 21, 2011.
9. Hall MA. Rethinking safety-net access for the uninsured. N Engl J Med 2011;364(1):7-9.
10. Redlener I, Grant R. America's safety net and health care reform—what lies ahead? N Engl J Med 2009;361:2201-4.
11. Griner PF. Payment reform and the mission of academic medical centers. N Engl J Med 2010;363(19):1784-6.
12. Seigel M. Medicaid cuts will make things worse. In: The Forum (7A). USA Today, Tuesday 19, 2011. p. 7A.
13. Kirch DG. A word from the President: the coming collision between US graduates and GME slots. AAMC Reporter; 2011. Available at: http://www.AAMC.org. Accessed July 21, 2011.
14. Orszag PR, Emanuel EJ. Health care reform and cost control. N Engl J Med 2010;363(7):601-3.
15. Iglehart JK. Implementing health care reform—an interview with HHS Secretary Kathleen Sebelius. N Engl J Med 2011;364(4):297-9.
16. Karpf M, Lofgren R, Perman J. Commentary: health care reform and its potential impact on academic medical centers. Acad Med 2009;84(11):1472-5.

17. Iglehart JK. The ACO regulations—some answers, some questions. N Engl J Med 2011;364:e35(1)–(3).
18. Kastor JA. Accountable care organizations at academic medical centers. N Engl J Med 2011;364:e11(1)–(3).
19. Berkowitz SA, Miller ED. Accountable care at academic medical centers—lessons from Johns Hopkins. N Engl J Med 2011;364:e12(1)–(3).
20. American Hospital Association Press Release. CMA underestimates the investment needed to create an ACO. Available at: http://www.aha.org/aha/press-release/2011/110513-pr-aco.html. Accessed July 20, 2011.
21. Berenson RA. Shared savings program for accountable care organizations: a bridge to nowhere? Am J Manag Care 2010;16(10):721–6.

Gastroenterologists and Accountable Care Organizations

Michael Komar, MD[a],*, Robert Smith, MD[b], Eileen Patten, BA[c]

KEYWORDS

- Accountable care organization • Gastroenterology
- Health care reform • Patient protection and affordable care act
- Medicare

WHY ACCOUNTABLE CARE ORGANIZATIONS?

On March 23, 2010, President Barack Obama signed the Patient Protection and Affordable Care Act into law, signaling the beginning of an effort to reorganize and restructure health care for Medicare beneficiaries. This law was aimed at correcting 2 of the most critical issues with the United States health care system: unduly spending and inconsistent quality of care. The United States spends more than $2.4 trillion on health care. Overall, the United States spends $3000 to nearly $5000 more per capita on health services (**Fig. 1**) and nearly twice as large a percentage of the gross domestic product than comparable countries worldwide, including Canada, the United Kingdom, and New Zealand.[1]

High health care costs threaten the sustainability of Medicare and the affordability of health insurance in general. Furthermore, despite these huge differences in health care spending, the United States falls significantly behind in measures of performance, including quality of care, efficiency, access to care, equity, overall health of patients, and adoption of integrated information technology.[2] Among those receiving Medicare in the United States, research has shown that, on average, regions with *higher* per beneficiary spending actually produce a *lower* quality of care and patient satisfaction. In other words, quality and cost are not intrinsically linked, and it may be possible to simultaneously improve the quality of US health care while decreasing expenditures.[3,4]

The authors have nothing to disclose.
[a] Geisinger Health System, 100 North Academy Avenue, Danville, PA 17822-2111, USA
[b] Adult Liver Transplant Program, Geisinger Health System, 100 North Academy Avenue, Danville, PA 17822-2111, USA
[c] Geisinger Health System, University of Michigan, 100 North Academy Avenue, Danville, PA 17822-2111, USA
* Corresponding author.
E-mail address: mkomar@geisinger.edu

Gastrointest Endoscopy Clin N Am 22 (2012) 39–49
doi:10.1016/j.giec.2011.08.004
1052-5157/12/$ – see front matter © 2012 Published by Elsevier Inc.

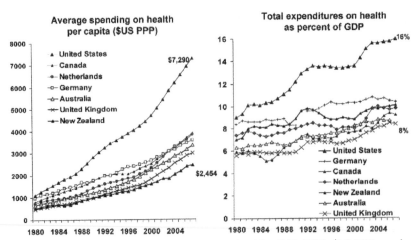

Fig. 1. International comparison of spending on health, 1980–2007. $US PPP, purchasing power parity. (*Data from* Organization for economic cooperation and development. OECD health data. Paris: OECE; 2009.)

Why does US health care lag in almost all measures of performance when spending exceeds comparable countries considerably? Part of the problem driving the high costs in the US health system, in addition to the greater use of hospital services, specialists, and diagnostic tests, is the burden of fragmented care with attendant waste and duplication. Furthermore, the current fee-for-service payment system rewards quantity of care rather than quality. Another factor driving spending stems from a minority of patients covered under Medicare and Medicaid who are responsible for 64% of the costs. Opportunities to lower spending include the avoidance of unnecessary hospitalizations, reducing rates of readmissions, expanded efforts to decrease hospital-acquired infections, and adding infrastructure for both preventative care and palliative care.[5]

In order for the US health care system, particularly the public health insurance programs, to sustain through the aging of the baby boomer generation and beyond, it is imperative that our nation finds some way to lower spending and amend wasteful practices that rise from the fragmentization and disorganization of the current system. In the federal government, one proposed solution uses health information technology and payment reform to better integrate and coordinate care, thus, allowing for a greater focus on quality of treatment over an episode of care. The medium for these changes comes in the government's recommendation to form accountable care organizations (ACOs).

WHAT DOES THE PATIENT PROTECTION AND AFFORDABLE CARE ACT SAY ABOUT ACOs?

In addition to extending coverage to millions of Americans through Medicaid and other mandates for health insurance coverage, the Affordable Care Act laid out mechanisms for the health care industry to reorganize to meet increased demand, improve quality of care, and lower costs.

In section 3021 of the act, the Center for Medicare and Medicaid Innovation was created to "test innovative payment and service delivery models to reduce program expenditures ... while preserving or enhancing the quality of care furnished to individuals."[4] In other words, this new component of the Centers for Medicare and Medicaid

Services (CMS) was given the significant task of selecting new models of payment and delivery of care aimed to maximize efficiency and quality of care.

Payment Schemes

ACOs are not a panacea but one of several complimentary initiatives within health care reform. Another area of health care realignment under the Affordable Care Act includes strategies for payment reform with reimbursement models that emphasize care for an overall population of patients. The act includes a provision that shifts payment away from fee for service and toward fee for performance or comprehensive payment, such as bundled or global payments. Fee-for-service payment has been targeted as fostering the application of unnecessary or wasteful testing and procedures that emphasizes quantity of care over quality, driving the hefty cost of health care higher.[1] The act sets up pilot programs to test the suitability of bundled payment schemes.

Although the traditional fee-for-service method of payment allocates a predetermined sum for individual tests or procedures, with bundled payments, a single fee is paid to cover the scope of services over an episode of care, which the act tentatively defines as beginning 3 days before hospitalization and continuing through 30 days following the patient's discharge.[6] Several health systems have already implemented such a payment scheme. For example, under Geisinger Health System's ProvenCare, all services—preoperative evaluation through rehabilitation—associated with certain surgeries, such as coronary artery bypass surgery, are covered for up to 90 days following the procedure by a single payment, regardless of any complications that may occur. It is possible that this form of bundled payment could extend to gastroenterological care, such as the management of hepatitis C.[1]

Coordination of Care

Another major area of focus in the Affordable Care Act is the coordination of care. The act sets the stage for the future development of ACOs. The ACO program is scheduled to go into effect January 1, 2012. ACOs are local networks of providers that are accountable for quality, cost, and overall health outcomes of a population of patients. They are voluntary networks that can be started by primary care physicians, hospitals, or other health care organizations; although specialists are not eligible to develop an ACO of their own, they will be allowed to participate. To achieve better coordination of care, it is widely anticipated that a greater emphasis will be placed on primary care and patient-centered medical homes. This, along with the expanded use of health information technology (HIT) and electronic health records (EHR) to improve care coordination, should lead to improved care at a lower cost.

OVERVIEW OF THE ACO MODEL
Qualifications

Requirements for starting an ACO include a formal legal structure responsible for the distribution of shared savings, a minimum of 5000 beneficiaries, an adequate number of primary care physicians to attend to this population, and submission of a 3-year plan. A proposed ACO would also have to prove their capability to promote evidence-based medicine, report on quality and cost data, implement HIT to manage EHR, and coordinate care among a team of professionals over the continuum of patient care.

If an ACO were accepted into the program, it would then be eligible to receive a percentage of Medicare savings per year if they met quality and cost-saving benchmarks.[7,8] The benchmark would consist of how much it cost to pay for Medicare fee-for-service patients assigned to an ACO over the previous 3 years, on average. The ACO will receive between 50% and 60% of the savings if expenses are less over the agreement period and other quality measures are also met. However, if Medicare pays more than the calculated benchmark, then the ACO may be responsible for a portion of the loss.[9] These quality and cost standards are still under negotiation, and recommendations from a range of interested parties regarding these measurements and the overall ACO structure are currently being considered.

Leadership

A key consideration for the development of ACOs is who will take the lead in forming them: hospitals or physicians? Although it is likely that both will take place, these different avenues would come with unique challenges and changes for the health care system in the areas that adopt them.

If hospitals are to take on the predominant role in forming ACOs, they need to shift focus away from the current business model of providing acute inpatient care, imaging, laboratory, and procedures to outpatient care, preventative care, and the overall coordination of care with the physicians they assume under their new health care model. The operational impact of decreased admissions, studies, and procedures on near-term revenue would likely subsume to more gradual long-term shared savings if the goals are met.

In areas where physicians take the lead in forming ACOs, there will be different challenges. Predominant among these would be a change in culture whereby long-standing competition among individual physician groups would have to succumb to a new mission of cooperation and collaboration. Furthermore, physicians may be resistant to a change in organization that would make them more accountable to oversight, require significant capital investment risk, and potentially lower their salaries because the anticipated savings that would come from better coordination of care would arise largely from avoiding tests, procedures, and hospitalizations. How to divide the shared savings among primary care physicians and specialists could also prove problematic.[5]

3-Tiered Entry

Following the acceptance into the ACO program, not all groups would be equally prepared to immediately enter into the requirements because US hospitals and physician groups have varying levels of existing integration among practitioners, information technology capabilities, and other key factors necessary to fulfill the standards of a full-fledged ACO. Therefore, health policy specialists have proposed 3 levels of ACOs, and an ACO could enter the program at any of these 3 levels and proceed according to their assimilation to the new system.

Level I or shared-savings ACOs would bear no financial risk but they would be eligible for shared savings if they met specified quality measures and savings targets. At this stage, the entry-level organization would be responsible for establishing a legal and managerial foundation, reporting administrative data indicating performance measures, gathering a sufficient amount of primary physicians to serve a population of 5000 Medicare beneficiaries, and developing an infrastructure for adequately attending to primary, inpatient, and outpatient care.

Level II or partial-capitation ACOs would take on some risk for spending more than the prescribed benchmark but would also be eligible for a greater proportion of payback on savings. Although level I ACOs would likely remain on a fee-for-service payment scheme, level II ACOs might begin transitioning into bundled payments or other comprehensive payment arrangements. In addition to the requirements under level I, level II ACOs would be responsible for more detailed reporting of performance, including measurements of patient satisfaction and chronic disease outcomes, as well as more comprehensive financial reporting standards.

Level III or fully capitated ACOs would take on both the most risk and the most potential rewards. These organizations would likely already have an integrated model of care and sophisticated system of electronic health recording in place. At level III, an ACO would be paid in large part or even fully through capitation or bundled payments, with significant bonuses based on success. In addition to the level I and II requirements, these organizations would need to make elements of EHR and patient reports available for use by the public and health insurance agencies as well as even more comprehensive financial reporting. To reiterate, if the care provided by an ACO costs less than Medicare predicts, the ACO will receive a share of the savings as a bonus payment. However, the rule also includes financial penalties if an ACO misses its targets. ACOs will also be required to withhold 25% of any bonuses it receives as an escrow to cover future potential losses.[9]

Although specific standards may vary, this 3-tiered plan allows for organizations at all levels of preparedness to enter into the ACO track and progress as they gain the infrastructure, skills, and experience to take on a greater role. This point is important because not all regions would be equally prepared to begin operating as ACOs because of the lack of collaboration within existing health care markets coupled with the few hospitals and physician practices with adequate HIT in place, which are essential core requirements.[8,10,11]

SPECIFIC ACCOUNTABLE CARE MODELS ALREADY IN EXISTENCE

Several existing models of health care organization would be ideal for the transition into an ACO status because of their patient-centered and accountable organizations, reliable systems of EHR records, or compensation strategies. Those most likely to be eligible for an entrance in the system that resembles the level III model are integrated delivery systems and multispecialty group practices, which have already established an infrastructure compatible with the ACO model.[8]

In an integrated delivery system, there are usually 1 or more hospitals melded with a primary and specialty physician practice under unified leadership. Core strengths include, at a minimum, an advanced EHR, a commitment to provide coordinated care, and, in some cases, a health insurance plan. Systems operating under the integrated delivery system model include Geisinger Health System, Intermountain Health System, and Kaiser Permanente.

Likewise, multispecialty group practices, such as Cleveland Clinic, Marshfield Clinic, and Mayo Clinic, that usually own or have a strong affiliation with hospitals, are equally well positioned given similar infrastructure, leadership, and access to capital for start-up costs, which may be considerable.

Other types of practice arrangements that could begin the process toward becoming more accountable for cost and quality, although probably at a lower level of ACO entry, include physician-hospital organizations (which sometimes function similarly to multispecialty group practices), independent practice associations, and virtual physician organizations (joining distant practices through the use of technology). Virtual physician organizations, in particular, would be ideal for rural areas whereby obtaining a patient base of 5000 necessary for ACO formation may be more difficult.[8]

WHAT WILL IT TAKE FOR SUCCESSFUL IMPLEMENTATION?

Adjusting to a new organizational and payment scheme will not be an easy transition. Because the ACO program is entirely voluntary (for both providers and patients), it is important that the government and other interested parties take every step to ensure that health care providers, who often tend to be resistant to change, are not dismayed by quality measures and cost savings that seem too difficult to achieve. This process requires realistic financial, clinical, and reporting goals that the aforementioned 3-tiered system could help to define and moderate for health systems with various levels of preexisting integration during the transition to ACO status.

Furthermore, quality benchmarks that will be used to determine shared savings earnings must be carefully considered and developed for each specialty. In the current proposal, only 1 of 65 measures that would be used to assess quality of care, colorectal cancer screening rates, is applicable to the practice of gastroenterology specifically.[12] One positive step that the Center for Medicare and Medicaid Innovation took was formally accepting recommendations from interested parties that will assumedly be used to develop the final quality benchmarks. The American Gastroenterological Association, for example, worked with the American Medical Association-sponsored Physician Consortium for Practice Improvement, National Quality Forum, and the CMS to develop validated clinical measurements and then built a reporting mechanism, the Digestive Health Outcomes Registry, which is specific to the practice of gastroenterology. They have submitted this, as well as other recommendations on CMS's 429-page proposal, to be considered in the finalization of ACO guidelines.[7,13]

Because only physicians and hospitals will be eligible to form an ACO, the role of specialists must be clearly laid out. The current proposal states that specialists would be able to participate as joint-venture partners or contracted participating providers. Specialists, unlike primary care physicians, would be able to join with multiple ACOs. A system of coordination and integration of specialists, therefore, must be determined, and patients with chronic conditions, such as end stage liver disease and inflammatory bowel disease, for whom gastroenterologists provide primary care services must be taken into consideration.[13]

Finally, it is imperative that a system of support is created to help participating hospitals and physician groups transition into cohesive units with the necessary infrastructure. To form an ACO, an organization would have to restructure legal and financial issues while potentially dealing with the task of acquiring an expanded staff of physicians and an increased number of patients. On top of this, ACOs would have to teach their staff a new system of organization and reporting, alter practitioner behaviors to become more cost-efficient and quality sensitive, foster teamwork among practitioners who formerly may have competed for business, implement and train staff to use an EHR systems, provide a foundation for reporting clinical and financial performance, and establish leadership able to foster and maintain these developments.[11] For some health systems, several of these tasks are already realized or in progress, but for many, these are hurdles that will require a great deal of patience, guidance, and money. For example, because it was estimated as recently as 2008 that only 21% of the physicians in the United States have access to a basic EHR system (which the Centers for Disease Control and Prevention [CDC] defines as including "patient demographic information, patient problem lists, clinical notes, orders for prescriptions, and viewing laboratory and imaging results") and only 4.4% have access to a "fully functional" system (for which the CDC adds the following requirements: "medical history and follow-up, orders for tests, prescription and test orders sent electronically, warnings of drug interactions or contraindications, highlighting of out-of-range test levels, electronic images returned, and reminders for guideline-based interventions"), this could incur a huge cost for implementation and training on organizations trying to gain ACO status, even considering stimulus money directed at developing these systems.[14,15] Adequate monetary and technical support for these transitions could lessen the burden. It has been suggested, for example, that current health systems operating under ACOs could take on a leadership position for newly developing ACOs and this service could be compensated in the form of a bonus or a greater payment of shared savings.[8]

OPPORTUNITIES FOR SAVINGS

The Health and Human Services Secretary Kathleen Sebelius has said ACOs could save Medicare $960 million in 3 years, but some experts doubt the financial feasibility for the health care organizations themselves.[16–18] Some point to the Physician Group Practice Demonstration, a pay-for-performance test of Medicare in which they selected 10 highly compatible physician groups to run a trial program that basically mirrors the proposed ACO format. Although all groups managed well in improving quality of care, only 2 of the groups were able to cut costs enough to benefit from shared savings in the first year of this program; by the third year, only half were successful in reaching the objectives necessary for a part of shared savings.[17,19]

Although the trial was not successful in reducing costs across the board, it does show that cost savings and quality improvement are possible.[12] There are multiple ways the ACO program presents opportunities for saving. On the most basic level, integrating care and focusing on the continuum of care rather than isolated instances will reduce costs that arise from care fragmentation in the fee-for-service model. Some areas of savings could include reducing duplication of services by more than 1 physician, reducing hospital readmissions that are more frequent when patients are not properly followed after discharge, and lowering the amount of late-stage complications by generating greater infrastructure for preventative care.[4,20]

Furthermore, the payment initiatives set forth have the potential to generate savings by making practitioners accountable and responsible for the amounts of costly tests and procedures they order. Under the current fee-for-service payment system, it is in a practitioner's best interest, or at the very least it is not discouraged, to order multiple tests because it may incur a greater payoff.[1,20] By focusing on quality instead of quantity, bundled or capitated payments hope to reign in wasteful spending and make providers accountable for their spending. In fact, with the shared savings programs and several other bonuses that have been suggested, physician groups and hospitals would be rewarded for implementing policies and practices that reduce costs.

Finally, the proposed provision to eventually require ACOs to publicly report data about their performance and finances will make hospital systems more accountable for the reasonable pricing of services. In addition, greater transparency will require ACOs to demonstrate that they are improving the quality of their care and not rationing delivery of care to keep costs low by neglecting to perform costly tests or procedures at the risk of their patients' health outcomes, as some may fear.[4,21]

CHALLENGES OR POTENTIAL DOWNFALLS

Certainly there are several challenges, and maybe even downfalls, to proceeding with the ACO model as proposed. Some of them were discussed earlier, in addressing the challenges of successfully implementing an ACO. However, there are some more macro issues that may be of concern.

There has been some apprehension, for instance, about the free-choice provisions that would remain in place if ACOs were established, allowing Medicare patients to freely choose what physicians and specialists they prefer to see. Just as the ACO program is voluntary for health systems, it is also voluntary for patients. Although Medicare beneficiaries will be assigned to ACOs based on primary care attendance, they will not be tied down to that ACO's services. As a result, it may be difficult to track quality of care or determine responsibility for quality or costs of care if patients do not remain under the care of a single ACO for the entirety of an episode of care or over the span of several episodes.[22]

In addition, there is concern that merging groups of physicians and potentially hospitals could create a setting in which competition is diminished, particularly in less-populated areas. This situation could also pose a significant problem for the private sector because market concentration has been attributed to the rising costs of health insurance.[23]

Finally, there are some who think that the proposed health care reform is neglecting a necessary step regarding reducing health care spending, that is, reforming tort law, which would in effect decrease the cost of defensive medical practices. A major challenge in assessing the true effects, both direct and indirect, of tort and medical malpractice on health care spending is the lack of clear evidence as to how much defensive medicine costs and the difficulty in measuring this practice. As a result, the issue of tort reform is an area of much debate; certainly some point to the costs of conducting unnecessary tests and procedures to ensure protection in the event of a lawsuit as a key factor in the burdensome cost of US health care, but others claim that the amount spent is minimal, about 2% of health care costs, and would not contribute to significant savings.[24,25] According to the Congressional Budget Office, placing a cap on noneconomic damages at $250,000, a cap on punitive damages at $500,000, and shortening the statute of limitations for filing lawsuits would yield an estimated savings of $54 billion over 10 years, a relatively modest sum when considering that the total Medicare and Medicaid spending is $992 billion for the current fiscal year.[26,27] Medical errors likely have a much greater impact on total annual spending.

SPECIFIC IMPACT ON THE PRACTICE OF GASTROENTEROLOGY

A shift to patient-centered ACO models could affect those who practice gastroenterology in a variety of ways. However, there is some uncertainty about the current precise impact, including how the process of specialists referrals will change in an ACO model and whether specialists referrals will decrease in an effort to reduce costs.

Currently, colorectal cancer screening is the only measure applicable to the practice of gastroenterology in the 65 quality standards required for ACOs to receive shared savings.[12] Although additional measures may be added to these standards, gastroenterologists can expect to see an increase in the rates of colorectal cancer screenings as a result. However, the new act has also given the Secretary of Health and Human Services Kathleen Sebelius and, in the future, the Independent Payment Advisory Board the power to determine reasonable reimbursement for health services and revalue them if they think they are too high. An increase in the numbers of colonoscopies could encourage them to reconsider and revalue the service, reducing reimbursement.[28]

More generally, the transition to the ACO model will lead to increased use of HIT, improved collaboration and coordination of care, and a greater focus on transparency. Extended office hours, in addition to greater use of physician extenders to improve access, will be needed to reduce costly emergency department visits. For example, to lessen emergency department visits, hospitalizations, and 30-day readmissions, there will need to be improved access to care, particularly providing more availability during traditional after hours and on weekends. This improvement could also include greater use of palliative services (eg, for patients with decompensated cirrhosis who are not candidates for liver transplantation). The development of patient-centered medical homes for patients with chronic gastrointestinal disorders (eg, inflammatory bowel disease) or chronic liver disease also seems likely.[4]

Finally, changes in the overall structure of health care delivery could mean changes in how one meets with patients. For example, in an effort to reduce costs and better coordinate care, new models of care, such as group visits for common conditions or e-visits for conditions that do not require on-site care, may become more common. Furthermore, with an increase in patients overall, practitioners may need to more heavily use nurse practitioners or physician assistants for more routine and straightforward cases.[4,11]

In addition to the revaluation of certain services, health care reform may mean salary reductions in the health care industry across the board. Although not directly explicit in the law, the overall goal of reducing health care costs and revaluing the services of primary care physicians could have an effect on salaries, particularly for specialists.[23] Furthermore, if ACOs are encouraged to reduce the number of referrals to specialists and manage certain services at a primary-care level, this would slow the flow of referrals to specialists, including gastroenterologists.

IMPLICATIONS FOR PATIENTS WITH CHRONIC GASTROINTESTINAL ILLNESS

Within the practice of gastroenterology, there are several groups of chronically ill patients who would probably benefit from some type of coordinated multidisciplinary care that would take personal responsibility and accountability for their ongoing care. The name typically used for such a care model is the patient-centered medical home.

Basic characteristics of such a care model are that it usually exists within a hospital or group practice structure; it involves physicians that specialize in the care of such patients; it can and does usually involve midlevel providers, nurse managers, and could also include dieticians and social services; and has affiliation with local home nursing services. Such care models make themselves available on short notice with expanded hours for regular checkups and consultations, which can either be through email, telephone, or clinic visit, or provide early identification of conditions that may lead to hospitalization or other emergency services with preemptive treatment. The use of evidence-based clinical guidelines, as well as maintaining an updated EHR, are required tools to successfully implement a patient-centered medical home.

One example is pre-liver transplant, peri-liver transplant, and post-liver transplant care. Patients who are listed for liver transplant initially undergo a multidisciplinary evaluation that includes the transplant surgeon, medical hepatologist, midlevel providers (both surgical and medical), social services evaluation, nutrition evaluation, and also financial services. Patients who are actively listed for transplant are then followed in a comprehensive fashion with frequent visits and with a designated nurse coordinator who is both accessible to patients and proactively contacts patients to coordinate all visits that are done before and after transplant.

This model could be expanded to gastroenterology at large to include patients with inflammatory bowel disease, treatment of chronic hepatitis C, and nontransplant candidates with end stage liver disease.

Potential benefits of a patient-centered medical home model can include a decrease in emergency visits, fewer hospitalizations, and savings in cost per patient per month to varying amounts depending on the populations studied. Other countries, such as New Zealand, use this model to a very high degree.[29]

FINAL THOUGHTS

For many, the path to the ACO model will require a substantial change in culture, significant cost for setting up the legal and information technology infrastructure, expanded use of EHR to lessen the fragmentation and duplication of services, payment reform, and a renewed emphasis on primary care and patient-centered medical homes. Successful implementation will require many changes, and it is essential that adequate support is given to providers throughout this process if the program is to gain widespread approval. In the restructuring of the health care system, it is critical that patients are well served, and patient-satisfaction measures, particularly regarding access and different mechanisms of care, including greater use of physician extenders, group visits, and e-visits, will be required to ensure patient cooperation and a high quality of care.

By changing the way it pays, under the ACO rule, Medicare is encouraging a new model for health care delivery to simultaneously bend the cost curve and improve quality, hoping that successful examples will become models for an increased field of ACOs and health care savings across the board. As a new business model, ACOs could fail if they are not able to assemble the management or information technology required, successfully meet the 65 quality measures, or generate the savings required to make a profit. The concept, although well meaning and ultimately necessary, could falter in its current form if adopted by too few to make a meaningful difference. This concern remains significant because even high-performing group practices, including Geisinger Health System and Dartmouth-Hitchcock, have signaled reservations about the ACO proposed rule, noting that the risks may be too high and the incentives too difficult to achieve.[22] However, regardless of whether the upcoming ACO program flies or flops, it is critical that some type of health care reform is performed if we are to assure sustainability in Medicare and the US health care system in the years to come.

REFERENCES

1. Dorn SD. United States health care reform in 2009: a primer for gastroenterologists. Clin Gastroenterol Hepatol 2009;7(11):1168–73.
2. Davis K, Schoen C, Schoenbaum SC, et al. Mirror, mirror on the wall: an international update on the comparative performance of American health care. New York: The Commonwealth Fund; 2007.
3. Baicker K, Chandra A. Medicare spending, the physician workforce, and beneficiaries' quality of care. Health Aff 2004;W4:184–97.
4. Lowell KH, Bertko J. The accountable care organization (ACO) model: building blocks for success. J Ambul Care Manage 2010;33(1):81–8.
5. Kocher R, Sahni NR. Physicians versus hospitals as leaders of accountable care organizations. N Engl J Med 2010;363(27):2579–82.
6. US Congress. H.R. 3590, 111th cong.: patient protection and affordable care act of 2010. Available at: http://www.govtrack.us/congress/bill.xpd?bill=h111-3590&tab=reports. Accessed May 25, 2011.
7. Kosinski LR. AGA assumes task of deconstructing ACO proposed rule and what it means for GIs. AGA Washington insider blog. 2011. Available at: http://agapolicyblog.org/. Accessed May 25, 2011.
8. Shortell SM, Casalino LP, Fisher ES. How the Center for Medicare and Medicaid Innovation should test accountable care organizations. Health Aff 2010;29(7):1293–8.
9. Medical shared savings program: accountable care organizations highlights of proposed rule. American Medical Group Association; 2011.

10. Fisher ES, Shortell SM. Accountable care organizations: accountable for what, to whom, and how. JAMA 2010;304(15):1715–6.
11. Shortell SM, Casalino LP. Implementing qualifications criteria and technical assistance for accountable care organizations. JAMA 2010;303(17):1747–8.
12. Berwick DM. Launching accountable care organizations—the proposed rule for the Medicare shared savings program. N Engl J Med 2011;364(16):e32. Available at: NEJM.org. Accessed May 31, 2011.
13. American Gastroenterological Association. Top 10 things GIs should know now about ACOs. 2011. Available at: http://www.gastro.org/advocacy-regulation. Accessed May 13, 2011.
14. Hsiao C, Beatty PC, Hing ES, et al. Electronic medical record/electronic health record use by office-based physicians: United States, 2008 and preliminary 2009. Washington, DC: Centers for Disease Control and Prevention; 2009.
15. Berkowitz SA, Miller ED. Accountable care at academic medical centers—lessons from Johns Hopkins. N Engl J Med 2011;364(7):e12. Available at: NEJM.org. Accessed May 31, 2011.
16. Kennedy K. Federal plan would streamline Medicare: HHS proposal could save $960M over three years. USA Today 2011. Available at: http://www.usatoday.com/. Accessed June 6, 2011.
17. Haywood TT, Kosel KC. The ACO model—a three-year financial loss? N Engl J Med 2011;364(14):e27. Available at: NEJM.org. Accessed July 20, 2011.
18. Berenson RA. Shared savings program for accountable care organizations: a bridge to nowhere? Am J Manag Care 2010;16(10):721–6.
19. Centers for Medicare & Medicaid Services. Medicare physician group practice demonstration: physicians groups continue to improve quality and generate savings under Medicare physician pay-for-performance demonstration. Washington, DC: Department of Health & Human Services; 2010.
20. Goldsmith J. Analyzing shifts in economic risks to providers in proposed payment and delivery system reforms. Health Aff 2010;29(7):1299–304.
21. Fisher ES, McClellan MB, Bertko J, et al. Fostering accountable health care: moving forward in Medicare. Health Aff 2009;28(2):w219–31.
22. The accountable care fiasco: even the models for health reform hate the new HHS rule. Wall St J 2011. Available at: http://online.wsj.com. Accessed July 20, 2011.
23. Greaney TL. Accountable care organizations—the fork in the road. N Engl J Med 2010;364(1):e1. Available at: NEJM.org. Accessed May 31, 2011.
24. Hermer LD, Brody H. Defensive medicine, cost containment, and reform. J Gen Intern Med 2010;25(5):470–3.
25. Studdert DM, Mello MM, Brennan TA. Defensive medicine and tort reform: a wide view. J Gen Intern Med 2010;25(5):380–1.
26. The economics of U.S. tort liability: a primer. Washington, DC: Congressional Budget Office; 2003.
27. Elmendorf DW. CBO's analysis of the effects of proposals to limit costs related to medical malpractice ("tort reform"). Washington, DC: Congressional Budget Office; 2009.
28. Oh J. Six ways healthcare reform and ARRA will impact gastroenterology. Becker's ASC review 2010. Available at: http://www.beckersasc.com/. Accessed May 13, 2011.
29. Schoen C, Osborn R, Doty MM, et al. Toward higher-performance health systems: adults' health care experiences in seven countries, 2007. Health Aff 2007;26(6):w717–34.

Electronic Medical Records and the Gastroenterologist

Lawrence R. Kosinski, MD, MBA, AGAF

KEYWORDS

• Electronic Medical Record • Electronic Health Record
• Gastroenterologist

The development of the electronic medical record (EMR) has been an evolving process over the last 30 years, occurring in phases based on the availability of technology and the changing requirements of payment systems. As a result of the recent changes imposed by the Patient Protection and Affordable Care Act (PPACA), this is an age of disruptive innovation in health care[1] in which the business model is changing from a fee-for-service, volume-based system to a risk-based, fixed payment value system. Although it was written before the PPACA[2] as part of the American Recovery and Reinvestment Act (ARRA),[3] the Electronic Health Record Incentive Program has established new standards for what an EMR will need to be in the future.[4] The changes imposed by the program facilitate the changes that are imposed in the PPACA. This article reviews the regulations imposed by this legislation and describes what the electronic health record (EHR) of the future will look like as a result.

MEANINGFUL USE

On February 17, 2009, President Barack Obama signed public law 111-5, the ARRA, a stimulus bill intended to lift the American economy out of recession. An important component of the ARRA is the Health Information Technology for Economic and Clinical Health (HITECH) Act,[5] created in an effort to stimulate the medical community to accept and incorporate EHRs into their practices and to use these applications to promote best practices, with a national health information network as the desired end result. Meaningful use (MU) changes the way clinicians work.[6]

VISION

The vision of the HITECH Act is to enable significant and measurable improvements in population health through a transformed health care delivery system.

The author has nothing to disclose.
Illinois Gastroenterology Group, 745 Fletcher Drive, Elgin, IL 60123, USA
E-mail address: lkosinski@msn.com

giendo.theclinics.com

PRIORITIES

The priorities of the HITECH Act are as follows:

1. To improve quality, safety, and efficiency, and to reduce health disparities
2. To engage patients and their families
3. To improve care coordination
4. To improve population and public health
5. To ensure privacy and security protections for personal health information (PHI).

DEFINITION OF MU

MU is described in the Act as the use of "Certified EHR technology in a meaningful manner"; electronic exchange of health information to improve the quality of care, such as promoting coordination of care; and reporting on clinical quality measures (which will become more stringent over time).

Thus, to comply with MU, an EP must be using a certified EHR that shows the ability to share information with others involved in the care or management of the patient; one that must have the ability to transmit quality data to central registries.

THREE PILLARS OF MU

Thus there are 3 pillars to MU:

1. The use of a certified EMR
2. Participation in health information exchange (HIE)
3. Reporting of quality metrics to appropriate agencies.

BENEFITS AND PENALTIES

To incentivize providers to comply with MU, the HITECH Act provides financial incentives to eligible providers (EPs) who comply with the standards described in the Act. They are shown in **Table 1**. Each EP who complies with MU in the required time period (defined later) will be eligible to receive a total of $44,000. Those who do not comply will ultimately have at least a 3% reduction in their reimbursements that will continue indefinitely.

Table 1
HITECH act provider incentives

Adoption Year	Maximum Payment ($)							PFS Penalty
	2011	2012	2013	2014	2015	2016	Total	
2011	18,000	12,000	8000	4000	2000	0	44,000	—
2012	—	18,000	12,000	8000	4000	2000	44,000	—
2013	—	—	15,000	12,000	8000	4000	39,000	—
2014	—	—	—	12,000	8000	4000	24,000	—
2015	—	—	—	—	—	—	—	−1%
2016	—	—	—	—	—	—	—	−2%
2017+	—	—	—	—	—	—	—	−3%

Abbreviation: PFS, provider fee schedule.

STAGES OF MU

A project of this size that requires such a major change in behavior cannot be implemented immediately. Therefore, MU will be introduced in 3 stages. Stage 1, which begins in 2011, is concerned predominantly with EPs capturing clinical data in an electronic format and initiating quality reporting. In 2014, stage 2 expands with the addition of decision support, and, in 2015, stage 3 adds clinical outcomes MU criteria (**Fig. 1**).

HIE

The second pillar of MU is HIE, which is the ability of each of our MU-certified systems to communicate with another equally certified system.[7] This communication is critical to the success of the program.

HIE is defined as the mobilization of health care information electronically across organizations within a region, community, or hospital system. It provides the capability to electronically move clinical information among disparate health care information systems while maintaining the meaning of the information being exchanged. The goal of HIE is to facilitate access to, and retrieval of, clinical data to provide safer, more timely, efficient, effective, equitable, patient-centered care. HIE is also useful to public health authorities to assist in analyses of the health of the population.

How will HIE change practices? It will bring structured data elements into practices and allow the transmission of similar data to others outside a practice. Examples include the incorporation of structured laboratory data into EMRs. Complete blood counts are no longer presented as faxed documents. The values are instead entered in an EMR for hemoglobin, hematocrit, red blood cells, white blood cells, mean corpuscular volume, and so forth, which allows changes to be charted and patterns of change analyzed for every element.

HIE will also improve the communication of clinical information between providers. Patient visit data will be transmitted in a structured format called Continuity of Care Records (CCRs)[8] and Continuity of Care Documents (CCDs).[9] CCRs and CCDs allow clinical information exchange between and among primary care physician (PCPs) and specialty care physician (SCP). More importantly, because they are in a common format, the information is automatically incorporated into the EMR of the recipient. This process occurs seamlessly between practices even if they use different EMRs.

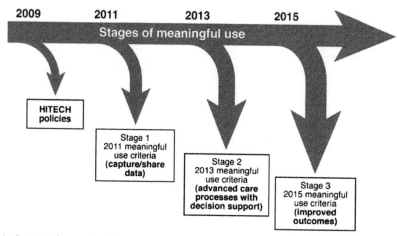

Fig. 1. Stages of meaningful use.

QUALITY MEASURES REPORTING

The third and final component of MU is quality measures reporting, and this is the most revisionary element. For purposes of the requirements under sections 1848(o)(2)(A)(iii) and 1886(n)(3)(iii) of the Act, clinical quality measures are defined to consist of measures of processes, experience, and/or outcomes of patient care, observations, or treatment that relate to 1 or more quality aims for health care, such as effective, safe, efficient, patient-centered, equitable, and timely care. Through this reporting, the Centers for Medicare and Medicaid Services (CMS) is beginning the move to value-based practice. A set of core quality measures has been developed that all providers will be required to report.

MU is expected to accelerate the conversion of the medical records present in all doctor's offices to digital data that can then be leveraged to improve the quality of medical care and lower its cost.

THE EMR AND ITS COMPONENTS

Clarifying the differences between an EHR and EMR is frustrating at times because so many people use the terms interchangeably. The CMS refers to the EHR because it represents the legal record containing confidential health and billing information drawn from the patient record and sent electronically to them for reimbursement. As a result, most federal agencies within the US Department of Health and Human Services, Social Security Administration, Office of People Management, and Veterans' Administration reference this system as an EHR.

However, vendors consider the software they sell to you to be the electronic version of a paper record that contains not only physician notes but also nursing notes, laboratory results, imaging reports, pathology reports, family and social history, and treatment plans. Therefore, they refer to their software as EMR. To help provide clarity to the discussion, the difference between EMRs and EHRs must be described. The following definitions have been developed by major authorities in health information technology.

EHR

As defined by the Healthcare Information and Management Systems Society (HIMSS),[10] the EHR is a longitudinal electronic record of patient health information generated by 1 or more encounters in any care delivery setting. Included in this information are patient demographics, progress notes, problems, medications, vital signs, past medical history, immunizations, laboratory data, and radiology reports. The EHR automates and streamlines the clinician's workflow. The EHR has the ability to generate a complete record of a clinical patient encounter (as well as supporting other care-related activities directly or indirectly via interface) including evidence-based decision support, quality management, and outcomes reporting.

Documentation of Patient Encounters

The components of a patient encounter include the following:

- Chief complaint
- History of present illness
- Past medical and surgical history
- Endoscopy history
- Family history
- Social history

- Review of systems
- Physical examination
- Assessment
- Plan
- Orders.

All of these elements must be documented on initial visits and must be at least referenced on most return visits. Although most of these elements can be entered into today's EMRs using picklists and dropdowns, the history of present illness is unique in that it must allow for flexibility in composition. This flexibility is accomplished in multiple ways including typing, voice recognition, use of macros, point-and-click options, and dictation.

The gastrointestinal (GI) EMR has a unique component, the endoscopic history. Clinicians need to know what endoscopic procedures were performed, when and for what reason, and the result.

Order Sets

Current MU-certified EMRs have the ability to create order sets that link a set of orders to a diagnosis, which is not only an efficient way to enter them but also provides for a more uniform style of practice in large groups. This method is essential for quality management and performance improvement and is discussed later. It also allows for the more efficient use of extenders.

The Endoscopy Report Writer

A major proportion of the services provided by gastroenterologists today are in the form of endoscopic procedures. Accordingly, the information produced by these services must be recorded and reported in a uniform fashion. The format of the endoscopy report has been worked out and has been reported by Lieberman.[11]

According to this guideline, the report must include the following fields:

- Patient demographics and history
- Assessment of patient risk and comorbidity
- Procedure indication(s)
- Procedure: technical description
- Findings
- Assessment
- Interventions
- Unplanned events
- Follow-up plan
- Pathology.

These essential components should be incorporated in all endoscopy reports. Endoscopy reports have traditionally been documents that record the details of the procedure that was performed. Through the use of a uniform set of formatted fields, these reports can be the tool that is used to refine the performance of procedures. Registries like the American Gastroenterological Association (AGA) Digestive Health Registry have been created by the societies to host and compile these metrics. Like all physicians, gastroenterologists will eventually be profiled based on the reporting of quality outcome metrics, the results of which will then drive reimbursement for their services.

Endoscopic Images

Most endoscopy reports also either include or reference endoscopic images that are obtained during the procedure. These images are captured and usually stored on a separate server. The EMR then must hold a script that allows it to access these images and incorporate them into the report. This access requires interfaces to be created from the endoscopy software and the EMR.

Pathology Modules

GI endoscopists also have a need for access to pathology reports. If the practice uses a commercial pathology company, then an interface is necessary that will send demographic information to the pathology company and receive report fields in return. If the practice has its own captive pathology company, it may or may not use a separate laboratory information system, which will require an interface as well. If the EMR is used for processing the pathology, then templates can be created within the EMR itself. Regardless of the structure, structured pathology data are essential for quality monitoring of issues like adenomatous polyp capture rates.

Patient Portals

A patient portal is a tool that allows a secure tunnel in the Internet to provide an interactive continuum of care between the patient and the physician, facilitating effective electronic communication and clinical data exchange.

Most portals contain standard features such as appointment requests, prescription renewals, and transmission of documents and forms. Other features of portals include importing referral documentation, and automated interviews that allow patients to complete their own history before the physician encounter. Customized disease and health management plans are also facilitated, based on the patient's input to the provider, who can then track, measure, and adjust plans. A portal integrates real-time clinical and administrative workflow among providers, hospitals, and patients.

In addition, a message can be sent to a group of patients identified for a medication recall, for a new service to help a chronic condition, or those due for tests or follow-up visits. Through a patient portal, messages are automatically addressed, encrypted for security, and sent to the targeted patients.

This is the future of physician-patient communication.

MOBILITY

Most gastroenterologists see patients in a variety of locations including hospitals and ambulatory surgical centers (ASCs). However, these locations are usually away from the physician's main office where the patient management system (PMS) and EHR are located, which creates issues in everyday practice. Every procedure performed in an ASC requires a timely history and physical examination. Clinicians therefore need access to their EMRs to accomplish this. The management of hospital inpatients often requires access to the clinical information stored in EMRs. Likewise, when clinicians are on call and have patient interactions, these must be recorded in EMRs for clinical as well as medical-legal purposes. These interactions all require real-time access.

The solution for this is to make use of Web-based tools either on personal computers (PCs) or handheld devices like smartphones or pads.

The major issues here include:

1. Real-time access to the data
2. Security of the communication

3. The ability to enter as well as receive data
4. Access to additional tools (eg, Performance Quality Rating Scale [PQRS]).

Real-time Access

Today, every communication between a physician or the nursing staff and the patient must be recorded. This requirement means that clinicians need to have the ability to connect to EMRs whenever it is required. This ability is especially critical in the group practice setting where one physician may be covering another, on call for another. Web-based access to EMRs allows for this type of communication.

Security

The security of the communication is critical. The Internet itself does not provide the level of security necessary for secure communication. One of the solutions for this is a connection called the Virtual Private Network (VPN), which creates a secure tunnel within the Internet that is password protected and encrypted. This protection adds the security necessary but requires an extra login and password that the user is required to enter.

Another means of safe communication is through the use of terminal server (TS) technology. The Microsoft Windows TS is a server program running on its Windows NT 4.0 (or higher) operating system that provides the graphical user interface of the Windows desktop to user terminals that do not have this capability themselves. Such terminals include the low-cost NetPC or thin client that some companies are purchasing as alternatives to the autonomous and more expensive PC with its own operating system and applications. The reserves a part of the server for each licensed user who then only needs to use a remote desktop application to access the full functionality of the EMR from wherever it is being accessed. Security is maintained and access is complete.

All of these features can be accessed using Web-based smart phones or pads. Data are in real time and security is maintained as long as the network is secure.

Another popular means of establishing secure real-time communications is through the use of active server pages (ASP), which create an application that sits on a Web server and communicates with 1 or more databases. ASP brings an application to the user that is accessible wherever there is Web access, and allows a safe, secure access to the databases that communicate with the ASP application. ASP applications are common in online services like banking. This technology is the basis of the so-called cloud where applications no longer reside in PCs but exist on a Web-based server. Once there, they can communicate with databases that are located elsewhere; this is the future of computing.

Choosing an EMR

The selection of an EMR can be a daunting task.[12] Currently there are more than 250 companies that sell EMRs. This number will undoubtedly decrease over time as consolidation occurs in the industry. How does the user choose? The first essential issue to consider is whether the software is MU certified. Only certified EHRs should be considered as viable choices. Once the field has been narrowed in this fashion, the other essential features for a GI practice need to be considered, such as GI-specific templates and an endoscopy report writer. Whether the software can be customized is a critical feature because clinicians need to customize the templates to their specific needs. What is the company's capability for service? Will they be responsive?

One of the most important steps in choosing an EMR is to find a champion within the practice, usually a physician, who will embrace the process and advise the rest of the physicians in the practice. Demonstrations of each EMR are critical. These demonstrations take time and focus, so a champion is essential.

QUALITY IMPROVEMENT

As discussed earlier, HIT can build a foundation for quality improvement (QI). CMS considers that the QI produced through the HITECH Act and MU will be an essential factor in the future control in the cost of Medicare and Medicaid. The success of health care reform relies on limiting the variation in the care that is provided. By limiting variation in care and promoting better adherence to evidence-based medicine, the overall cost of health care will be easier to control.

Most clinicians practice with a knowledge base that has been built in medical school and in postgraduate training, but continually refined through continuing medical education either in the form of journal articles or educational sessions. However, the fields in which clinicians practice are continually expanding the requirements of their knowledge base. In addition, this is a period of shared outcomes in which clinicians are expected to report results into registries that are large databases composed of fields of clinical data. The hope is that, by accumulating this data, it can be leveraged to improve decision making.

Registries

In order for this to be accomplished, the data has to be transmitted to the registries in real time and seamlessly so that it does not interfere with the provision of medical care. To do this, common formats are required. With the marked heterogeneity in EMR data structure, this is difficult. In time, these common fields will be formatted and data will be transmitted unencumbered.

Once there are large clinical data repositories, it will be possible to create standards for performance and then benchmark providers against these standards. The main goal of benchmarking is not to identify outliers but to provide a means for providers to conform to the standards by showing them how they compare with their peers.

Clinical Decision Support Tools

The essential next step after registries is the creation of clinical decision support (CDS)[13] tools, which are vehicles to feed back assistance in decisions to providers. They will not only assist physicians who are outliers to conform to standards, but will also assist even the best physicians to improve the value of their work. Ultimately, standards will tighten and the bell curve of performance will tighten. Levels like 6 σ may never be reached, but medical practice will become less variable.

Real-time CDS tools will supplement and potentially replace some of the previous tools of continuing medical education because they will be in real time and narrowly focused on the specific clinical situation in which the physician is practicing.

These tools will be even more useful to the less trained physician like the PCP or the physician extender like the Nurse Practitioner or Physician Assistant. CDS tools will allow care for certain conditions (eg, IBS) to be provided by the less trained professionals and still maintain the same level of quality, which will be essential to cost control.

Order Sets

Originally referred to as cookbook medicine, order sets have become an essential component of the implementation of EMRs. They allow us to create a standard set of orders for each clinical diagnosis that is encountered. They not only improve quality, they enhance efficiency and help control cost. In addition, they help define the state of the art.

Order sets are integrated with knowledge databases so that clinical references can be accessed in real time to confirm the accuracy of each component of the order set.

PUTTING IT ALL TOGETHER AROUND RISK AND VALUE

The age of risk-based value-driven reimbursement has begun. This age will create a myriad of challenges, starting with a change in the drivers of income. Traditionally, physicians have been reimbursed for volume, not value, but this has now been reversed. One of the most significant challenges in moving to value is to find/create the metrics for quality. These metrics have not yet been adequately defined. The metrics must satisfy the following equation:

$$\text{Value} = \frac{\text{Quality}}{\text{Cost}}$$

Because Quality = Service + Outcome, value can now be defined as:

$$\text{Value} = \frac{\text{Service} + \text{Outcome}}{\text{Cost}}$$

Metrics for service can easily be developed through patient satisfaction surveys. Cost is easy to calculate as well. The challenge is in metricizing the outcomes. Values for this need to be developed over time. CMS is working in this space in conjunction with the National Quality Forum (NQF). As they endorse and implement measures for PQRS, the ratio of encounters that meet the standards can be used as a metric.

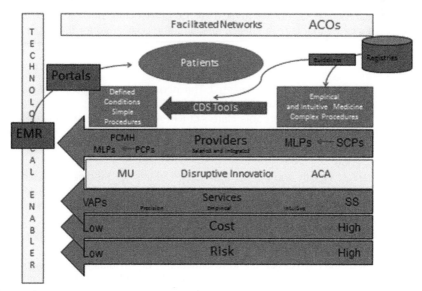

Fig. 2. The new structure. ACA, Accountable Care Act; ACO, Accountable Care Organization; CDS, clinical decision support; MLP, midlevel providers; PCMH, patient centered medical home; SCP, specialty care physician; SS, specialty shop; VAP, value-added process.

Fee-for-service medicine is being replaced by value-based medicine, which will create an environment of reimbursement based on fixed salaries combined with bonuses driven by scores on a balanced scorecard of production, financial, patient satisfaction, and quality reports.

How will EHRs help? See **Fig. 2.**

In order for providers to control risk, cost needs to be controlled. This control requires transforming specialty shop (SS) services like complex consultations into value-added processes (VAPs).

With VAPs, protocols and guidelines will guide the provider. EMRs will pull data from registries and drive the creation of detailed practice guidelines that will then support the development of CDS tools. These tools will allow less trained health care participants to participate in the care model at higher levels than they do today. Thus, intuitive medicine will move toward more precision-based services. The disruptive innovations of the PPACA and MU will facilitate the movement of services from high-price specialists to PCPs and midlevel providers, thereby lowering cost and maintaining quality.

Without the data management and CDS tools provided by the EHR, this will not be possible.

SUMMARY

HIT has gone through a long maturation process driven by changes in technology and payment systems. This is an age of disruptive innovation in health care in which the business model is changing. Fee-for-service, volume-based systems are being replaced by fixed-fee, value-based systems. One of the major facilitating forces behind this change has been the development of the EHR, which is providing the medical community with the ability to have real-time quality metrics. These metrics will drive the development of Web-based CDS tools that will transform the current peer-review–based rules of practice with an eclectic fluid environment of continuous quality measurement and improvement. It will be challenging, but the result will be a health care system that is high quality, efficient, and positioned for the future.

REFERENCES

1. Christensen CM, Grossman J, Hwang J. The innovator's prescription: a disruptive solution for healthcare. New York: McGraw-Hill Books; 2009.
2. Patient Protection and Affordable Care Act ("PPACA"; Public Law 111–148).
3. Pub L No. 111–5. American Recovery and Reinvestment Act of 2009. Available at: http://www.gpo.gov/fdsys/pkg/PLAW-111publ5/content-detail.html. Accessed February, 2009.
4. Department of Health and Human Services: Centers for Medicare & Medicaid Services. 42 CFR Parts 412, 413, 422, and 495, CMS-0033-F, RIN 0938-AP78.
5. Hitech Act. Available at: www.hhs.gov/ocr/privacy/hipaa/administrative/enforcementrule/hitechenforcementifr.html. Accessed February, 2009.
6. Kosinski LR. Meaningful use and electronic medical records for the gastroenterology practice. Clin Gastroenterol Hepatol 2010;8:494–7.
7. Federal Register/Vol. 76, No. 5/Friday, January 7, 2011/Rules and Regulations.
8. American Society for Testing and Materials (ASTM) E2369 - 05e1 Standard Specification for Continuity of Care Record (CCR).
9. The Continuity of Care Document: Changing the Landscape of Healthcare Information Exchange. Corepoint Health; 2011.

10. EHR – Based Quality Measurement & Reporting: Critical for meaningful use and health care improvement. Chicago (IL): Health Information and Management Systems Society; 2010.
11. Lieberman DA, Faigel DO, Logan J, et al. Assessment of quality of colonoscopy reports: results from a multi-center consortium. Gastrointest Endosc 2009;69(3 Pt 2):645–53.
12. AGA Field Guide: Selecting and Implementing Electronic Medical Records for your GI Practice. AGA Institute Press; 2009.
13. National Quality Forum (NQF), Driving Quality and Performance Measurement—A Foundation for Clinical Decision Support: A Consensus Report. Washington, DC: National Quality Forum; 2010.

A Letter to Fellows: Transitioning From Training into Practice in Uncertain Times

Rahul S. Nayak, MD, MBA

KEYWORDS

- Gastroenterology • Health Care Reform
- Patient protection and affordable care act

TRANSITIONING FROM FELLOWSHIP TO PRACTICE

You have nearly finished the formal part of your training. Until now, each step has been clear: finish college, attend medical school, apply for residency, and then apply for and complete a fellowship. Given the competitive nature of each of these steps, most people do not choose their paths; each of us is chosen. This final step, the transition from fellowship to practice, is the least discussed step, but it is your opportunity to make some important choices.

This article discusses 6 steps that can help structure your job search and provide some tools and tips to help you understand the process. It also discusses trends that define the market.

Two important legislative health care bills were passed during your fellowship: the Patient Protection and Affordable Care Act and the Health Care and Education Reconciliation Act. Although the legislative portion was passed, the lines of federal regulations have yet to be defined. Despite their implications for your job search, their major effect is to create uncertainty regarding the ultimate law and the day-to-day ramifications of the regulations. Regardless, although there are many potential areas of impact on gastrointestinal (GI) practices, the law has changed the job search in several ways.

1. Uncertainty may lead to reticence in expanding a GI practice for many groups. Many GI practices are small businesses and, in this time of economic uncertainty and increased unemployment, some patients are losing their coverage or putting off preventive services.[1] This slowdown and the continued uncertainty makes further investments in expansion seem more dangerous. Thus, practices that

The author has nothing to disclose.
Gastroenterology, Southwood, The Southeast Permanente Medical Group, Kaiser Permanente, 2470 Mt Zion Parkway, Jonesboro, GA 30236, USA
E-mail address: jainyak@gmail.com

Gastrointest Endoscopy Clin N Am 22 (2012) 63–75
doi:10.1016/j.giec.2011.08.011
1052-5157/12/$ – see front matter © 2012 Elsevier Inc. All rights reserved.

may have been considering hiring are waiting to see when the economy is going to improve. Furthermore, the current controversy regarding health care reform is increasing the level of uncertainty in the market. Actively growing a practice based on a health care reform act that may be partially or fully repealed in 2 years has been giving many physicians pause and encouraging a wait-and-see attitude.

2. Consolidation of practices will accelerate and there will be fewer solo practitioners and small groups.[2] The push toward consolidation is in response to the increasing challenges of insurance company negotiations and the restriction of the capital market to make investments in ambulatory surgery centers and radiology services, and to seek greater economies of scale. This trend has even extended to more rural areas with larger practices expanding geographically to ensure a steady income stream.

3. Accountable care organizations (ACOs) may begin to define practice patterns (this is a caveat of issue number 2). The ACO is being positioned as a way to track the use of health care resources. One of the most significant impacts may be a change in the traditional fee-for-service model to a bundled payment system for care of disease conditions. The relationship of specialists to these organizations is not yet well defined, and every practice should have an active strategy regarding their participation in ACOs. However, changes will occur that will necessitate a change in the design and operation of the GI practice.[3,4]

4. An electronic medical record (EMR) is essential, not an option. In many ways, the EMR used to be a nice addition to a practice, but this is no longer true. The EMR is close to the heart of health care reforms, and practices should either have or be actively transitioning to an EMR. This transition represents a substantial financial as well as strategic commitment that will pose a challenge to many practices, especially smaller ones. After 2015, penalties for not participating in the EMR requirements start at 1% of Medicare fees, rising each year to a maximum of 5%.[5]

PRACTICES AT THE 10,000-FT LEVEL

Although health care reform will have an impact on the future of medicine in the United States, the opportunities for practice in gastroenterology remain diverse. There are several different practice opportunities and they are limited only by your own imagination. However, the current environment breaks down into some dominant practice models. There are positives and negatives to each of these models (**Box 1**; **Tables 1–5**).

Each of the models has multiple variations. There are several very large GI groups that have the advantages of a single-specialty practice and allow overheads to be spread among many people, thus reducing the cost per person. Hospital positions may provide stable employment; however, the autonomy of these positions is usually limited. Large multispecialty groups provide the comfort of a built-in patient referral system. However, decisions for the group are made at the board level, minimizing your independent impact on the group's day-to-day management, financial

| Box 1
Practice options |
|---|
| Solo |
| Single specialty |
| Multispecialty |
| Hospital employed |
| Academic |

Table 1 Solo practice model	
Pro	**Con**
Maximum flexibility in time	Coverage issues
Income directly linked to effort	Harder to access ancillary income
New technologies make it easier to control overhead/scheduling	New technology is expensive for 1 physician
Hire/fire, manage staff and practice	Managing practice takes away from patient care

distribution, and future. Academic practices may allow some combinations of clinical practice, research, teaching, and administration. Financial reimbursement may be reduced compared with private practice settings; however, protected time for research and teaching may exist. Combination of practice settings may also exist. Kaiser Permanente and Sutter Health are 2 examples that combine the advantages of a multispecialty practice and academics.

Practice variations are regional; in the northeast, the dominant type of practice continues to be smaller, single-specialty groups, whereas in the Midwest and South, very large groups often dominate the environment.

DETERMINING YOUR PRACTICE PREFERENCES
Step 1: Set Your Priorities

The first step to finding a good practice fit is to clearly define your short-term and long-term priorities. If you want to have total control of hiring/firing, strategic business decisions, and the color of the scrubs that your staff will wear, being an employee will not be a good fit. If living in an urban environment is the highest priority, then looking at a rural practice does not make sense.

I have found the following set of questions to be nearly universal in understanding what really matters to you.

Where do you (and/or your family) want to live?

This is the most important question that you have to answer, and it is the one that you should spend the most time on. You should plan to factor in your spouse's needs, other family members, weather, urban/rural settings, as well as personal comfort. The most challenging places to find available practice opportunities tend to be within the major cities. If you want to live in those areas, you must be prepared to make other compromises.

Table 2 Single-specialty (general) practice model	
Pro	**Con**
Coverage built in, shorter and more regular hours	You may disagree with coverage intervals or geography
More likely to be able to access ancillary streams	Partnership issues can be challenging
Share fixed costs across group	Decreased control over practice
Allows for GI-specific synergies	Benefits may require >5 practitioners

Table 3 Multispecialty practice model	
Pro	Con
No need to recruit patients or advertise	Loss of autonomy, more bureaucracy
Salary vs salary with production vs production	May not get access to ancillary income
Better care coordination between primary care physicians	Lower compensation
Call variable, hours generally shorter than solo	No control over staff

How much autonomy do you want to have?

If you want to run a small business, either start your own practice or join a small group practice, because this allows for maximum control over your practice and life. However, control does not equal freedom. In contrast, if you just want to see patients, do procedures, and then head home without a great deal of input into the operations of the practice, then the larger practices are for you.

Do you want to teach?

If the answer is yes, start looking at academic opportunities or large, well-established, multispecialty and group health practices. There are many institutions that provide teaching opportunities, so do not limit yourself to just major academic medical centers.

Do you like predictability?

There are many different ways to structure your day, and they break down into 2 basic models. In one model, you see patients in both the outpatient and inpatient setting. In the other model, you do all outpatient work except during discrete weeks when you cover the hospital, in which case you will be doing only inpatient work. Most larger groups have adopted the second model.

Do you like call?

Regarding call, it should be noted that not all call is the same. For instance, 1 in 4 first emergency room (ER) call from a busy hospital with a significant cirrhotic population is not the same as 1 in 4 call for a rural practice. In some practices, call represents the way that you get new patients; in other practices, patient volume is so great that it is not a relevant source. In addition, some practices ask that newer physicians take more call compared with senior partners as part of the sweat equity that is required to be partner eligible.

How much do you want to make?

This is the question that most people focus on first; generally, that strategy leads to short-sighted decisions. Putting an absolute number into hourly terms helps to

Table 4 Hospital/employed practice model	
Pro	Con
Set hours, set benefits	Loss of autonomy, increased bureaucracy
Familiar practice environment	No access to ancillary streams of income
No buy-in, maximum flexibility to move	No control over staff
Opportunities for administrative roles	Lower compensation

Table 5 Academic practice model	
Pro	**Con**
Research opportunities, teaching opportunities	Loss of autonomy, increased bureaucracy
Familiar practice environment	No access to ancillary streams of income, lower compensation
No buy-in, maximum flexibility to move	No control over staff
Freedom to specialize, teaching opportunities	Pressure to publish and be productive

understand what you are making. All the other aspects noted earlier must also be taken into account to make a well-rounded decision for both you and your family.

The following is an example of 2 potential salaried positions:

Practice 1: salary: $175,000
Practice 2: salary: $250,000

At first glance, practice 2 seems to pay most. However, see **Table 6** for a breakdown. Practice 2 makes less on a per-hour basis, based on a 48-week work year. However, thanks to your hard work of prioritizing your goals, you can now put this into context. If you need the additional $75,000 per year, and if practice 1 is not going to let you be any more productive than a 40-hour work week even if you want to, then practice 2 is going to be the best for you. The concept is to compare like with like as much as you can; just comparing salary in this setting does not tell you the whole story.

Your priorities may change as you work through the process, so do not be surprised if you have to come back to these questions a couple of times.

Step 2: Prepare

Having set your priorities, it is time to prepare for your new position applications by obtaining the necessary tools. The first step is to update your curriculum vitae (CV) and create a single-page resume. Most practices want a CV, but the process of creating a single-page resume helps to focus your experiences and may aide in guiding your priorities.

Highlight your unique experiences and skills, such as the extra month of inflammatory bowel disease (IBD) training at a center of excellence, or specialty training in endoscopic retrograde cholangiopancreatography/endoscopic ultrasound (EUS), motility, nutrition, pill cam, and liver experience; these are all things that can set you apart.

Using your CV, create a cold call script, introductory networking e-mail, cover letter, and thank-you letter. All of these share similar elements but can be used differently depending on the interaction and can be customized for each practice. These tools

Table 6 Salaried position breakdown		
Salary	**Hours Per Week**	**Hourly Salary ($)**
Practice 1: $175,000	40	90
Practice 2: $250,000	60	85

are often your first impression and should be carefully created to showcase your interest in the practice as well as why they should be interested in you.

Appendix A includes samples of all of these tools.

The final step of your preparation for your new position application is to create an organization tool for your search. This tool can take almost any form that works for you, but should include the elements in **Box 2**.

An example of a spreadsheet is given in Appendix B.

Step 3: Research and Network

There are many different sources of information to tap into, and some are better than others. Resources have recently been moved online, but there are many practices that do not have any real Web presence, and finding those practice opportunities takes work.

If you are limited geographically, starting with a simple Internet search will uncover many possible practices. In reviewing a practice's Web site, read anything listed under practice philosophy as well as the biographies of the physicians. Also study the business manager, and his or her background and experience.

Expand your online search to include visiting the Web site of the major societies as well as reviewing publications such as the New England Journal of Medicine or Gastroenterology. These sources allow you to review practice opportunities that are being advertised in these venues.

Box 2
Elements of a position application organization tool

Name of practice

Name of practice manager

Contact details of practice

Number of partners

Managing partner

Number of offices

Number of hospitals covered

Call schedule

Partnership

Ambulatory surgical center

Laboratory

Pathology

Date practice was contacted and how they were contacted

Who you spoke to

Date CV was sent

What follow-up have you done and dates when it was done

Response

Notes regarding personal connections to practice

Notes regarding interview impressions (best done immediately after interview)

Many of the best opportunities are gained from networking. Begin to actively reach out to your friends, residency connections, both residency and fellowship programs, as well as the device and pharmaceutical representatives who you have met and respect. College and medical school networks can also be useful because many of your former classmates may be located where you want to go.

A couple of notes: you do not need to be friends with someone to reach out to them to ask for help or opportunities. Often, a group connection, such as graduating from the same college or medical school, will catch someone's attention. See **Box 3** for some well-established rules when reaching out to people.

Although this is not an easy process to start, once you have done it a couple of times it becomes easier.

The art of the cold call

If you cannot find a connection to a practice that you are interested in, then sometimes you may need to pick up the phone and give them a call. Calling is stressful, and may make you feel like a telemarketer. However, done correctly, it can be an extremely effective way of getting noticed.

Before making the call, it is important to learn as much as you can about the practice that you are going to cold call, including research on their Web site and tapping into resources such as LinkedIn to obtain background information on the physicians. Next, practice your cold call script and pitch with friends until you are comfortable. It can take several tries to get it right and, even then, there will be some variation when you make the call as a result of being nervous. When you call the practice, ask to speak with the practice manager or the person who makes hiring decisions. After exchanging greetings, begin your cold call script.

There are 3 potential outcomes:

1. They want your CV
2. They are not thinking about hiring right now or had not considered it
3. They are not hiring.

Following up in all 3 cases with a cover letter/CV and thank-you note is a good idea. Circumstances change; if you get 1 of the last 2 answers, ask the manager if there is a good time to call back and check in and be willing to call back in a couple of months to see whether their response is different.

A special note about recruiters: headhunting firms can be a good source of information, but they are most often employed for practice opportunities that are considered less desirable. However, they represent a way of expanding your options, particularly if you do not have any connection to a geographic area that you are interested in.

Box 3
Rules for reaching out to people

1. Be clear about your connection and what it is you are looking for from them.

2. Asking for advice or guidance is an effective way to open a conversation.

3. Someone you reach out to will recommend another person to reach out to; always follow up this recommendation and send a thank-you note back to your contact.

4. Contact may be done via e-mail, phone, or in person. Be sure to include what your connection is to them as well as what information or advice you are seeking.

Step 4: Interview

Your networking and research has paid off and now the practice wants to interview you. Preparing for an interview is like any other aspect of your job search: it benefits greatly from some careful thought and a great deal of practice.

First, make sure that you have studied the practice's Web site, read the member biographies provided, and read their mission statement. The more that you know about the practice, the easier it is to have a conversation. Second, make sure that you know your CV thoroughly. If you have to answer a question about a research project that you used to pad your CV but are not that knowledgeable about, you could be in trouble. Third, few people are born knowing how to interview well. Recruit some trusted friends to help and work on some practice interview questions. For instance, you should not be surprised by the questions found in **Box 4**.

Make a list of questions that you want to ask the practice. Often, after asking a couple of questions about your CV, the next question a busy partner will ask is the dreaded, "So, what can I tell you about our practice?" Awkward silence is the worst response.

Evaluating a practice is more like beginning a long-term relationship and less like another 3-year stop you were used to during your training. In that context, your goal during the interview is to answer some key questions for yourself (**Box 5**).

There are several different ways to establish the answers, but following your instincts can be the most important. Capture your impressions in your spreadsheet immediately after interviewing.

Try to talk to everyone in the practice; it will help you develop a better understanding of the practice. Liking the physician partners is great, but remember that the day-to-day staff are the people you will actually be working with most closely. Making a positive impression on them may sway the partners in your favor rather than another qualified candidate.

For most practices, you represent a large investment in time, energy, and resources. Recruiting and supporting a new physician is a major process, and most practices want to invest in a long-term partner.

Step 5: Weighing Up Your Options

Ideally, you will have more than 1 offer. Thanks to the work that you have done, you should have an informative spreadsheet that breaks down the pros and cons of each practice that wants you. Return to your list of priorities and resist the temptation to adjust them because of the offers. Measure each practice according to your core priorities and let your informed intuition decide.

There are some red flags to be aware of when evaluating a clinical practice:

1. No ladder: if a practice has several partners in their 60s and several physicians in their early 30s, watch out; the junior members are probably brought in to create

---

Box 4
Potential interview questions

Why do you want to join this practice?

What is appealing about our practice?

Do you have any special interests?

Tell me about your strengths/weaknesses?

Why do you want to be in this geographic area?

Box 5 **Self-evaluation questions**
Do I want to work here for a while? Do I fit within the culture? Do people seem happy? Do I like the physical space of the office?

revenue and then transitioned out after a couple of years. Further, when the senior members retire, the junior members may be obliged to buy them out, possibly at exorbitant rates. In contrast, if a practice has a couple of physicians in their 30s, 40s, 50s, and 60s, this practice hires with the intent to make you a partner.

2. Complicated contracts: contracts are for both your protection and the protection of the practice. Although you do not know how to write a contract, your potential practice should. Any contract of more than 3 to 5 pages is becoming complicated. Any contract of more than 10 pages may be ridiculous. Complicated contracts contain clauses and subclauses that you need to read; unfortunately, many people do not. This situation is dangerous. At a minimum, the noncompete clause, the consequences of breaking the noncompete, productivity definitions, salary expectations, path to partnership, benefits information, and ways you can get released from your position should be well defined and understood. Some shorter contracts provide those details in other attached documents. Make sure that you read and understand those supporting documents and bylaws as well.

3. Vague promises: this is a classic conundrum. You met the practice. You liked the practice. The practice told you verbally how your employment and future partnership would be designed. However, the written contract does not include those details. Always get it in writing. If the practice does not want to put it in writing, assume that it is not going to happen.

4. Sudden changes in the terms of the contract: this can happen for legitimate reasons. However, those reasons should be clear to you. If they are not, it is probably time to walk away.

Once you have narrowed an offer down, you will generally have to sign a contract. Before doing this, make sure that you have the contract reviewed by a lawyer. Not all lawyers have a skill set that is adequate for this situation. You need a good labor lawyer with experience in physician contracts, in the relevant state, and, ideally with gastroenterology experience. Often, people with this degree of experience are expensive. Given that you are committing 1 year of your life (possibly more) to this practice, spend the money to have your contract reviewed. There is still room to negotiate the contract terms at this point, but do not follow the same tactics you use to buy a car. The relationship between you and your new practice is going to be ongoing and should be positive.

Step 6: The First Year of Practice

See **Box 6** for a some general points on how to make the first year successful.

If things are not working out, make sure that you know why. If you do not, the same thing may happen again should you find another opportunity. Take some solace in knowing that many physicians leave their first job. You have a sought-after skill set and the freedom to move on. Health care is going through momentous changes

---

Box 6
Considerations for first-year success

1. Be someone who says Yes except when you should say No. An extra patient who needs to be seen in the office unexpectedly? Yes. Need some coverage? Yes. Want me to do something crazy that I have no experience doing? No.

2. Complications happen to everyone. Try not to put yourself in a situation in which a complication is likely.

3. Be friendly, open, and helpful.

4. Take care of your staff.

5. Take care of yourself and your family.

6. Find a niche that interests you and own it.

7. Do not buy a house for the first year of your new position.

---

and, in many respects, these changes are accelerating. Being open and willing to change is one of the most important attributes that you can cultivate. Consider this: 30 years ago, our specialty was more of an intellectual endeavor; with a few key changes in technological advances, it has become one of the most sought-after procedural-based careers in health care.

SUMMARY

The end of your training marks the beginning of your learning. Moving into practice is exciting, and there are good opportunities. Although there is still a great deal of uncertainty with the economy, you have a skill set that is in demand. By understanding your real priorities, being deliberate and organized in your search, and being willing to extend outside your comfort zone, you will find a practice that fits you. Remember that each person has an ideal practice. What may be ideal for your friend or colleague could be a disaster for you. Most importantly, choose your new practice setting with your eyes wide open, especially regarding new changes that are expected with health care reform.

REFERENCES

1. Zaldivar, Ricardo. Recession slowed health care spending. Available at: http://www.msnbc.msn.com/id/40934441/ns/health-health_care/t/recession-slowed-health-care-spending/. Accessed August 29, 2011.
2. Allen, John. What Do You Think of Obamacare Now? Available at: http://www.gastro.org/mobiletools/policy-updates/734. Accessed August 29, 2011.
3. American Gastroenterological Association. What GIs Need to Know about Accountable Care Organizations. Available at: http://www.gastro.org/practice/practice-management/aga-think-tank/what-gis-need-to-know-about-accountable-care-organizations. Accessed August 29, 2011.
4. AMA. "What Health System Reform means to physicians and patients". Available at: http://www.ama-assn.org/ama/pub/advocacy/current-topics-advocacy/affordable-care-act/ama-comments-on-aca-regulations.page. Accessed August 29, 2011.
5. Lewis, Morgan. Physicians unconcerned about EHR penalties. Available at: http://www.modernmedicine.com/modernmedicine/Modern+Medicine+Now/Physicians-unconcerned-about-EHR-penalties/ArticleStandard/Article/detail/696497. Accessed August 29, 2011.

APPENDIX A: EXAMPLE LETTERS AND CONTACT INFORMATION
1. Cover Letter

GI Joe
  1904 Evergreen Avenue
  Evanston, Il 60203
  314 867 5309
  yojoe@yahoo.com
  Date
  Address
  Address
  Dear [X],
  I am entering the third year of my gastroenterology fellowship at the [X]. Although I have enjoyed my time in [X], my wife and I are planning on returning to the [X] to be closer to family and friends. [Insert your compelling reason to be in this area]
  During my gastroenterology fellowship at the [X], I have been exposed to a wide spectrum of diseases in gastroenterology and hepatology in a diverse patient population. By the completion of my fellowship I will be trained in colonoscopy, endoscopy, small bowel capsule endoscopy, 24-hour pH monitoring, and esophageal manometry. I believe these qualifications would be an excellent match for your practice.
  Thank you for your consideration. I will contact you next week.
  Sincerely,

2. Cold Call Script

1. Hello, my name is Dr [X]. May I please speak with the person/physician in charge of hiring/managing partner/CEO?
2. I am currently a GI fellow at [X]
3. I found your name through the Alumni network/personal connection/Web directory and would like to talk to you about your practice and any potential opportunities. Is now still a good time?
4. Ok great, well let me quickly start off by giving you some background about myself:
   a. I graduated from [X] (college)
   b. Attended medical school at [X]
   c. I then did my residency at [X]
   d. As I mentioned, I am currently a second-year fellow at [X]
5. My [Insert your reason for wanting to go the area: family, personal connections, deep desire to live in the area] and I am now pursuing private practice opportunities in the area.
6. I have read up on your practice and am extremely interested in finding out about opportunities with your group.
7. I was hoping you could tell me a little bit about your background, and more about the practice in general, as well as any general advice.

3. Initial E-mail Contact to Alum

Dear [X]
  My name is [X] and I found your contact information through the [X] Alumni Network.
  I graduated from [college] and with an MD from [medical school]. I have completed my internal medicine residency at [program], and I am currently a second-year gastroenterology fellow at [program].

I am exploring practice opportunities in [specific area] because [personal and compelling reason for moving to this area]. We are looking forward to moving back into the area where we have family and friends. I would welcome a chance to talk to you to get some advice on opportunities in [area].

Is there a good time for us talk later this week? I look forward to hearing from you.

Thanks,

4. Pharma E-mail Contact:

Dear [X],

Best wishes in the New Year. We have met several times at [program], and I am currently a second-year fellow there. I am exploring practice opportunities in [area].

I was hoping that you could give me the name of the representative for your company in that area or help me learn more about the various practices in the area. I have a copy of my resume that I can send to you or to any of your colleagues.

Because I have not made any concrete decisions about my career path, I hope that we can keep this as discrete as possible. I appreciate any help that you can provide.

Thanks for your time and I look forward to hearing from you.

Sincerely,

5. Examples of Second-level Questions (ie, Past the Initial Conversation or During the Interview)

I have some second-level questions, I enjoyed talking to you, so wanted to find out more details. Thanks for taking the time to speak with me.

Find out more about job:

How do you work clinic? Maybe 4 to 5 half-day clinic, 3 half-day sessions, hospital coverage fits in; perhaps rotating 1 week hospital. How many days per week clinic, how many days per week procedures?

How do nurse practitioners/PA fit in?

When do you see inpatients?

How long do patients have to wait to get into clinic?

How many procedures?

Breakdown?

How many on weekends, how many on nights?

Where are the procedures done?

Any procedures in office?

Future plans? In-office endoscopy? Ambulatory surgical centers (ASCs)? Radiology? Pathology? Other ancillary services?

Future trends? Population changes?

Who does hospital consults? How are they divided up?

Do you have an inpatient service or is it purely consultative?

Any macro trends?

How much liver disease?

How much IBD?

Does the hospital do transjugular intrahepatic portosystemic shunts?

Does the hospital have equipment for EUS?

Long-term plans for the practice?

Coverage?

Partnership

APPENDIX B: SAMPLE SPREADSHEET

State	Address	Name of Practice	Type of Practice	Alumni Connection	Pathology/ Radiology/ASC
CT	1450 Luminal Way www.gastro.org	Endo Kings	Single specialty	N	N
MO	4000 Villous Drive www.colyte.org	Everybody in	Multispecialty	Jeff Bloom	Y: radiology

Medical Practice Integration: Going Big in Private Practice

Kimberly M. Persley, MD, Rajeev Jain, MD

KEYWORDS

- Medical practice • Integration • Private practice
- Infrastructure

In 2009, according to an American Society of Gastrointestinal Endoscopy (ASGE) survey, 55% of gastroenterologists practice in groups of less than 6 physicians, 22% in groups of 6 to 10 physicians, and 15% in groups of greater than 10 physicians.[1] Individual and small groups are coalescing or integrating in response to the combination of financial and health policy pressures. In 2009 in the United States, there were at least 5 gastroenterology groups with more than 40 physicians and 50 groups with 10 or more physicians.[2] Data from the Community Tracking Study has identified 4 major reasons large, single-specialty groups form: (1) to have capital and scale economies to invest in practice infrastructure; (2) to gain negotiating leverage with health plans; (3) to gain reputation as a high-quality group; and (4) to gain professional management to deal with an increasingly complex business and regulatory environment.[3] This article reviews the rationale for gastroenterologists to integrate their practices to go big in private practice.

REASONS TO GO BIG
Practice Infrastructure

Various quality and performance initiatives are being implemented by health plans and payers that will link payment to documenting and reporting patient outcomes data. For example, the Tax Relief and Health Care Act of 2006 established a Physician Quality Reporting Initiative (PQRI), which increases payments by 1.5% to physicians who report information on specific quality measures to Centers for Medicare and Medicaid (CMS). PQRI now is termed the Physician Quality Reporting System (PQRS). Similarly, private health plans and large purchasers of health care are linking physician payment to pay-for-performance (P4P) measures. Gastroenterology practices need robust health information technology (HIT) or electronic medical records (EMR) to collect, track, and submit patient data and outcomes to receive the bonuses for PQRS and P4P measures. In the future, practices will be financially penalized for not reporting

Financial disclosure: Salix (speakers bureau), UCB (research), Abbott (speakers bureau).
Texas Digestive Disease Consultants, 8230 Walnut Hill Lane, Suite 610, Dallas, TX 75231, USA
E-mail address: kpersley66@aol.com

Gastrointest Endoscopy Clin N Am 22 (2012) 77–83
doi:10.1016/j.giec.2011.08.009
1052-5157/12/$ – see front matter © 2012 Elsevier Inc. All rights reserved.

quality data. The adoption of HIT/EMR is expensive and would generally be beyond the reach of many solo and small practices.[4,5] Generally, a large group is in a better financial position to raise the capital to acquire and deploy HIT. In addition, the economies of scale allow funding and development of ancillary service lines (eg, infusion centers, ambulatory endoscopy centers, pharmacy, and pathology) that can produce additional revenue streams to the large practice. A detailed discussion on the development of infusion services has been provided by Ancowitz and Shah.[6]

Negotiating Leverage

The ability of a large group to gain leverage in negotiating reimbursement has been the main reason cited for joining or creating a large practice group.[7] With mergers and consolidation in payers and hospitals, small practices and solo practitioners are at a disadvantage when negotiating with these large entities. For example, by 2003, the 3 largest insurance plans in 47 of the 50 states controlled more than 50% of the patient enrollment in those states.[8] Large practices with their negotiating leverage may be necessary to minimize the continued decline in reimbursement offered by payers. For example, in a study of large multispecialty physician practices in California, the more concentrated physician markets were able to charge higher prices to health plans because of their market power.[9] In addition, the negotiating leverage can lead to discounts in the cost of office infrastructure (eg, EMR, computers, and supplies).

Quality

All physicians desire to practice high-quality medicine; however, the Institute of Medicine reports a quality gap attributed to the growing complexity of science and technology, the increase in chronic conditions, a poorly organized delivery system, and constraints in the use of information technology.[10] In order to practice high-quality medicine and gain peer and patient recognition, gastroenterology practices need to identify and disseminate best practices while measuring patient outcomes and satisfaction against validated benchmarks.[11] Endoscopic quality measures have been proposed.[12–16] Participation in a clinical registry that seamlessly integrates into HIT/EMR (eg, American Gastroenterological Association [AGA] Digestive Health Outcomes Registry) can allow practices to perform continuous quality improvement to reach desired benchmark levels. In addition, large practices often have thought leaders or experts within the group who can assist in developing clinical decision support and critical pathways that are supported by guidelines. Effective implementation of these clinical tools is time consuming and often requires modification of HIT/EMR. The greatest obstacle can be physician participation.

Professional Management

A large practice needs professional medical practice management to deal with the increasingly complex business and regulatory environment in the United States. A professional medical practice management team can bring sound business principles and plans for practice marketing, operations, billing, collections, contracting, and growth. Physician leadership within the organization remain critical but a professional medical practice management team can allow physicians to focus more on medical rather than administrative issues.

PRACTICE TYPES

Today, physicians have multiple types of practice opportunities to consider. Many years ago, there were 2 practice options, academic or private practice. Times have changed. A graduating gastroenterology fellow today has the opportunity to choose from several different practice options (see article elsewhere in this issue). It is important that gastroenterologists look at their particular needs when assessing the ideal practice setting.

The most common practice types are described later with a brief description of each practice type with its lifestyle characteristics and perceived advantages/disadvantages.

Private Practice

In a solo practice, the gastroenterologist is the lone practitioner. Typically, the administrative and clinical staff is small. Therefore, the solo gastroenterologist must be highly organized and have good financial management skills and a willingness to accept financial risk. The solo gastroenterologist makes all the decisions and is in complete control of the practice. Patients see the same provider for every visit, thus creating a strong doctor-patient relationship.

A solo gastroenterologist may have to work long hours and have little time off. The financial risk tends to be higher in a solo practice than in other practice types. The overheads tend to be higher compared with group practices. Fluctuations in the economy may have a greater effect on the solo gastroenterologist. Despite these disadvantages and current trends in health care, there will always be gastroenterologists in solo practice but they will need to adapt to survive the changes in health care.

A solo practice may operate best in a rural area that cannot support a larger gastroenterology group. In other settings, offering a specific niche not offered by others in the community may also allow for success in a more urban setting.

In a group practice, patient care duties and physical space are shared among a group of physicians. A single-specialty group practice may be attractive because of several factors. A fixed cost of operating a practice is shared among the partners in the group. Partners can share on-call responsibilities, therefore affording a more controlled lifestyle. Days may be shorter and coverage is available, allowing for more free time outside the office. Many choose to join a group practice because of increased financial security and better lifestyle. There is often collaboration between partners, which can be helpful in making the difficult diagnosis. A group practice may allow for internal specialization. The clinical and professional strengths of the partners can help in creating a local gastrointestinal supergroup. Additional specialty training (eg, inflammatory bowel disease, hepatology) or expertise in certain procedures (eg, endoscopic ultrasound, endoscopic retrograde cholangiopancreatography) may be attractive to referring physicians and patients. Large groups can develop sophisticated management of patient populations or clinical service lines (see article elsewhere in this issue).

Large groups or megagroups are not for everyone. Disadvantages of large group and megagroup practice may include a decrease in autonomy and lack of equality. In large groups there is usually physician leadership that controls the governance of the practice. Personality conflicts may make it difficult to work with a large group. In simple terms, not everyone can get on well with other people. Some personalities do best when they are in charge. If someone is unable or unwilling to accept the administrative leadership recommendations, it could make an unpleasant environment for all of the partners. No one expects total agreement on every practice management issue, but there should at least be a shared mission and vision accepted by the partners. Another disadvantage of a large group or megagroup is lack of equality (real or imagined). Are all partners treated equally? Do some partners receive benefits not afforded to other partners? Is there a hierarchy among the partners? Problems may develop if compensation models seem biased or unfair. Is revenue split equally? Is there an equal opportunity to produce? Is there an opportunity to buy into an ambulatory surgical center? These are all important questions that should be asked when considering joining a large group.

In a multispecialty group, the gastroenterologist partners with nongastroenterologists. This entity may have internists, gastroenterologists, cardiologists, and rheumatologists working as a group. Multispecialty groups provide multiple patient services at 1 location and have the potential to negotiate favorable managed care contracts. This type of group includes an established patient referral pattern. There is less financial risk than in solo practice. Salary, benefits, vacation, and medical education time tend to be attractive. Gastroenterologists tend to have lower salaries compared with the single-specialty group practice.

These larger practices are associated with more bureaucracy. Loss of autonomy and decision making are the major disadvantages of this type of practice.

Employed Physician

The employee gastroenterologist works in a practice or department that is managed and owned by a larger entity. The gastroenterologist is an employee and compensated by the entity. This type of practice may be academic, public health (government), or in a hospital-based setting. The advantages of this practice type include a large referral network of practices, more effective managed care negotiations, and financial security. The larger entity assumes the financial risk. It is important that the larger entity is financially sound. The hospital will have a marketing strategy for the practice. It is important that there is agreement in the hospital marketing and the individual practice.

The employee gastroenterology practice is usually less lucrative compared with the single-specialty group practice. Income from ancillary revenue streams may not exist in this type of practice. There may be significant committee work in this type of setting. There may also be teaching responsibilities required in this type of practice.[17]

Locum Tenens

Locum tenens is also an option. In this setting, the gastroenterologist is employed by an agency to work for short periods from several weeks or months at a time. It gives the gastroenterologist the opportunity to try out the market in a certain area. This type of temporary employment may be ideal for some. The gastroenterologist has the ability to choose not only the practice geographic location but may also allow schedule flexibility. Salary is competitive and an agency typically picks up the cost of malpractice insurance. The physician generally does not receive health care coverage or retirement plan opportunities.[18]

PERSONAL CHARACTERISTICS

When considering going big, it is important to examine personal needs. Many gastroenterologists are interested in a work-life balance. Economic pressures may also be pushing gastroenterologists into big practices. There have been significant changes in health care in the last several years. Change is inevitable in life and in health care. In this changing environment, many decisions are being made based on fear and doubt. Is the decision to go big the result of uncertainty in what the future holds for the gastroenterologist? Making a decision based on fear of the unknown can result in regrets and disappointment when things do not work out as planned. Fear should not be the driving force when considering a change to a large practice option. There are many practice options for the practicing gastroenterologist; this could be the perfect time to examine the personal goals, financial needs, and professional vision. The answers to these questions may direct the gastroenterologist to the ideal practice.

Is a balanced work life important? If someone does not have an appetite for long hours and little free time, solo practice should not be pursued, because a large group may be the preferred option. Young children and other responsibilities outside medicine are factors that need to be considered when deciding on a practice option.

How much financial risk am I willing to take? With significant student loans and debt, many gastroenterology fellows may be risk averse and desire greater financial compensation. In larger groups, there may be lower operating costs per partner because of shared fixed overheads, higher reimbursements because of better contracts and access to a larger referral network. Most importantly from a physician compensation standpoint, a large practice may allow for the opportunity to benefit from ancillary or passive revenue streams.

What is my professional vision? A strong vision about a practice may not be shared with a large group. If unable to compromise with the vision, then a small practice may be the best option. A large group is a good option for those who enjoy collaboration with others. A specific interest within gastroenterology (eg, inflammatory bowel disease, liver disease, or advanced therapeutics) is likely to be easier to pursue in a large group. In a large group, the gastroenterologists interested in leadership positions can play a pivotal role in the management of the practice. New technologies and treatments, and participation in national guidelines and registries may be a professional vision. This vision would be difficult to pursue in a small or solo practice.

A big group is not for everyone. Possible loss of autonomy and identity, and decreased decision making are disadvantages of a large group. In a solo practice or small group, there is complete control of the management of the practice. The physician makes every decision, big or small. Some personality traits may make it difficult to join a big group. Some people need to be in control and loss of autonomy is not acceptable. Practice decisions made by others may be difficult to accept. If autonomy and decision making are important, then a small group or solo practice is probably a better option.

Taking the time to ask these questions about your personal needs and giving yourself truthful answers will make the decision to go big easier.

TIMING

Is there an advantage of going big immediately after fellowship? Are there any advantages of starting small and going big at a later time? Many new physicians change jobs or practice settings within the first 5 years after graduation, which suggests how difficult it is for physicians entering practice to envision the lifestyle, work-family balance, and requirements in a private practice setting. Therefore, it is important that graduating fellows do their homework regarding the practice types before making the decision to join a solo, small, or big practice. It is important to talk to former fellows and more established gastroenterologists when considering a practice option, especially when assessing the gastroenterology marketplace in a particular geographic location.

Many fellows consider joining larger groups on graduating. It is important to ask the right questions regarding compensation, road to partnership, workload, and access to ancillary income.

Is there ever a bad time to consider going big? What about gastroenterologists who are slowing down in their practices? They may be planning to retire soon and therefore production may be decreasing. It is important to look at the terms of group partnership before making the decision to go big. Is the overhead split equally among the partners, or does the overhead decrease as production decreases? Does the compensation/distribution model change if certain benchmarks are not met? What is the attitude of the other partners regarding the more seasoned gastroenterologists in the group? Are they thought to be an asset because of years or practice, experience, and contacts? Are they seen as a financial burden because of declining production? These are the questions that should be addressed before going big.

LOCATION

Location is extremely important when considering a change in practice types. Regional, state, and community factors have to be considered when deciding on a practice type. It is important to ask the following questions: does a particular group dominate in its marketplace? Is there competition in the area from other groups? What are these other groups like? Do the homework and find out what the practices are like in the area where you desire to practice. Large groups and megagroups tend to be found in more populated urban areas. It could be difficult for a solo practice or small group to compete in this setting. In locations saturated with gastroenterologists, referral patterns are usually set. Breaking those patterns in a solo or small group may be difficult.

In a rural setting, a solo practice or small group may do well. These smaller markets may not be able to support a large group.

REGULATORY ISSUES

In forming a large practice, the physician stakeholders need to comply with many regulatory issues. If a new entity or practice is being formed, the new physician organization will need to register with the appropriate local, state, and national authorities. In addition, the new large practice organization may need to obtain a new single-physician provider number from CMS as well as recredentialing with insurance plans. Most importantly, the large practice should consult with attorneys with specialization in medical practice mergers to comply with antitrust laws and other legal matters.

SUMMARY

Faced with the current economic conditions and impending regulatory requirements, gastroenterologists are coalescing to form large, single-specialty gastroenterology groups to maintain their financial viability and promote high-quality patient care. The time has come to go big in private practice.

REFERENCES

1. Littenberg G. Where will health care reform take GI practice? Gastrointest Endosc 2010;72(2):396–401.e392.
2. Bosworth T. Gastroenterologist trend toward larger practices. Gastroenterology and Endoscopy News, vol. 60. New York: McMahon Publishing; 2009.
3. Casalino LP, Pham H, Bazzoli G. Growth of single-specialty medical groups. Health Aff (Millwood) 2004;23(2):82–90.
4. Goldzweig CL, Towfigh A, Maglione M, et al. Costs and benefits of health information technology: new trends from the literature. Health Aff 2009;28(2):w282–93.
5. Lee J, Cain C, Young S, et al. The adoption gap: health information technology in small physician practices. Health Aff 2005;24(5):1364–6.
6. Ancowitz B, Shah SA. Infusion services in the gastroenterology practice. Gastrointest Endosc Clin N Am 2006;16(4):727–42.

7. Casalino LP, Devers KJ, Lake TK, et al. Benefits of and barriers to large medical group practice in the United States. Arch Intern Med 2003;163(16):1958–64.

8. Robinson JC. Consolidation and the transformation of competition in health insurance. Health Aff (Millwood) 2004;23(6):11–24.

9. Schneider JE, Li P, Klepser DG, et al. The effect of physician and health plan market concentration on prices in commercial health insurance markets. Int J Health Care Finance Econ 2007;8(1):13–26.

10. Institute of Medicine. Crossing the quality chasm: a new health system for the 21st century. Washington, DC: National Academies Press; 2001.

11. Brotman M, Allen JI, Bickston SJ, et al. AGA Task Force on Quality in Practice: a national overview and implications for GI practice. Gastroenterology 2005; 129(1):361–9.

12. Rex DK, Petrini JL, Baron TH, et al. Quality indicators for colonoscopy. Gastrointest Endosc 2006;63(Suppl 4):S16–28.

13. Baron TH, Petersen BT, Mergener K, et al. Quality indicators for endoscopic retrograde cholangiopancreatography. Gastrointest Endosc 2006;63(Suppl 4):S29–34.

14. Jacobson BC, Chak A, Hoffman B, et al. Quality indicators for endoscopic ultrasonography. Gastrointest Endosc 2006;63(Suppl 4):S35–8.

15. Cohen J, Safdi MA, Deal SE, et al. Quality indicators for esophagogastroduodenoscopy. Gastrointest Endosc 2006;63(Suppl 4):S10–5.

16. Faigel DO, Pike IM, Baron TH, et al. Quality indicators for gastrointestinal endoscopic procedures: an introduction. Gastrointest Endosc 2006;63(Suppl 4):S3–9.

17. Alguire P. Types of practices. 2011. Available at: http://www.acponline.org/residents_fellows/career_counseling/types.htm. Accessed July 11, 2011.

18. Darves B. Differentiating among medical practice settings. 2000. Available at: http://www.nejmjobs.org/career-resources/medical-practice-issues.aspx. Accessed July 11, 2011.

Gastroenterologists and the Triple Aim: How to Become Accountable

John I. Allen, MD, MBA[a,b,*]

KEYWORDS

• Triple aim • ACO • Accountable • Principal care

Whether or not accountable care organizations (ACOs) become a reality during the evolution of health care in the United States, they will force changes in the care of patients with complex or chronic diseases toward a more organized, coordinated model. Providers will be held accountable for outcomes, and reimbursement will move from a volume-driven model to one based more on demonstrable improvement in health value.[1–3] If physicians want to avoid being marginalized during this transition, they must present viable models of care that are evidence based and meet the needs of major stakeholders. Physicians must demonstrate that they are responsible stewards of health care resources who can achieve excellent patient health outcomes.[4,5] Berwick and colleagues[6] have defined this overarching goal of US medicine as the triple aim, which is to improve care of the individual, maximize health of a population, and reduce overall costs.

Gastroenterologists have an opportunity to assume a central role as managers of both medical care and health care resources for populations of patients with several chronic digestive diseases, including inflammatory bowel disease (IBD), gastroesophageal reflux disease (GERD), chronic liver disease, colorectal cancer prevention, and nutritional disorders among others. When specialists manage a population, this is termed principal care in contradistinction to primary care. As primary care providers (PCPs) are evolving their practices into patient-centered medical homes (PCMHs),[7] specialists can become patient-centered medical home neighbors (PCMH-N).[8] Here, patients with certain chronic conditions are comanaged by the PCMH and the

The author has no funding or support.
The author has no financial disclosures.
[a] Minnesota Gastroenterology PA, 5705 West Old Shakopee Road, Suite #150, Bloomington, MN 55437, USA
[b] University of Minnesota School of Medicine, Minneapolis, MN 55455, USA
* Minnesota Gastroenterology PA, 5705 West Old Shakopee Road, Suite #150, Bloomington, MN 55437.
E-mail address: jallen@mngastro.com

Gastrointest Endoscopy Clin N Am 22 (2012) 85–96
doi:10.1016/j.giec.2011.08.007
1052-5157/12/$ – see front matter © 2012 Elsevier Inc. All rights reserved.

specialty practice, but the responsibilities and communication expectations are clearly defined to maintain PCP-specialty coordination.[8] At times, some patients will identify the specialist as their principal point of contact with the medical system. Examples of PCMH-N can be found in oncology. As an example, when a cancer becomes the key health issue for patients, then the management of their health care would be transitioned to an oncologist.[9] Although this is uncommon in gastrointestine (GI), in a formal sense, the concept of principal caregiver is apparent in many current clinical practices and even can be introduced in a staged manner for those in traditional practices of any size.

As pointed out by other authors in this monograph, evolving practice into a principal care model will enhance patient outcomes and will allow to advance up the food chain of reimbursement (see articles 4 and 9 elsewhere in this issue). Achieving success will require physicians to focus on high-cost patients, coordinate care across multiple service sites, build practice infrastructure to support a chronic care model, increase office visit opportunities, reduce fragmentation, respond to the acute needs of patients, manage medicines more proactively, and provide appropriate preventive care.[10]

This article outlines a stepwise approach to managing a clinical service line. Minnesota Gastroenterology PA has implemented the initial steps of such a program. Minnesota Gastroenterology is a large, integrated, single-specialty practice in the upper Midwest. Several subspecialty areas of focus have been developed over the last 5 to 8 years, including IBD, esophageal disorders, and chronic liver disease. This monograph discusses the IBD program as it stands now and outlines future plans as we move aggressively into an advanced chronic care practice model. The author draws illustrations from other two other service lines to explain the hypothesis that an independent practice can provide a must-have clinical service that a regional ACO or health care system would find difficult to replicate within an employment model. Independent gastroenterology practices are decreasing in number, and many specialty practices are being purchased by hospital systems.[11] Although some high-profile physician-hospital organizations (PHOs), such as Mayo Clinic, Cleveland Clinic, Geisinger Health System, or Intermountain Health Care, can develop robust GI service lines, most PHOs do not have sufficient depth in their GI departments to provide the same level of expertise, geographic coverage, or coordination that can be achieved using the model described here. Practices that can embrace current imperatives to integrate care of complex patients and develop PCMH-N will become indispensable (and irreplaceable) for regional health care systems. Practices that remain focused factories of endoscopic procedures risk becoming simply a discounted commodity. Of importance, this model is scalable, that is, it does not require practices to be large and highly capitalized. What is needed is a patient-centered focus, a coordinated team of providers who can deliver the needed services in a timely manner, and a sufficient health information technology (HIT) to manage patients at a population level and extract clinical outcome data.

ESSENTIAL UNDERLYING PRACTICE INFRASTRUCTURE

Today, US health care is preoccupied with competition for market share, cost shifting, and cost reduction, all played out within a zero-sum game.[8] As articulated by Porter and Teisberg,[8] the right kind of competition will improve outcomes by incorporating 3 guiding principles: (1) emphasis on value for patients, (2) organization around medical conditions and care cycles, and (3) measurement of risk-adjusted outcomes and costs. Building an infrastructure within a GI practice to accomplish such a transition requires the following 7 steps (usually in this order):

1. Development of a strong physician-led governance in which the primary focus is on everyone together building a patient-centered practice.
2. Alignment of compensation and partners' philosophy with the mission and vision of the practice (usually meaning that production-based compensation must be modified to support program building and team-based care).
3. Building a robust HIT system that is capable of easy data entry, population identification (eg, all patients with IBD), registry function, action alerts, standard order sets, clinical decision support (CDS) tools, and other advanced information methodology.
4. Support of dedicated subspecialists with recognized disease-specific expertise (and ongoing continuing medical education).
5. Clinical care algorithms that define points of care transfer (PCP to specialist, general specialist to the IBD Care Team), evidence-based guidelines (with the capability of assessing compliance), and validated outcome measures.
6. Capability of resource identification (what is spent on the population) and Lean analytic capability.[12]
7. Development of the care team and infrastructure to provide acute care, urgent care, and chronic care.[13]

Although these steps seem daunting and will take time, small practices can accomplish most, if not all, aspects of a PCMH-N and examples have been published.[7] Large specialty practices have advantages with economies of scale, enhanced capital, the ability to cross-subsidize (many partners still performing colonoscopy, whereas others managing complex cognitive care), and other factors not found in small offices. The relative ease of information transfer, proximity of the needed services, and culture of cooperation advantage the multispecialty practices. Although current reimbursement does not favor a PCMH-N model, changes that will emanate from the Patient Protection and Affordable Care Act (PPACA) will change medical payments in a manner that will support this transformation. Other chapters in this monograph have outlined the key components of the PPACA as they relate to value-based payments and accountability (eg, chapters 1 and 9).

GOVERNANCE STRUCTURE, PARTNER COMMITMENT, AND COMPENSATION

The current governance structure of this practice includes participation in leadership roles and committees by a wide variety of physicians who understand that their contributions help support the larger practice goals and are not provided to further personal agendas. Most positions are volunteer, although leadership positions are compensated enough so that partners do not feel compromised economically when they assume leadership of this large corporation (more than 500 employees). Compensation demonstrates the practice commitment to physician leadership and the importance of these positions. Secondly, widespread participation in committees or Clinical Focus Groups assures of the depth of expertise needed to design robust programs.

Key committees determine how the practice delivers care, including the Operations Management Group and Clinical Focus Groups (eg, IBD), each of which reports to the Clinical Practice Committee. The Quality Committee provides improvement goals and performance measures. The Finance Committee defines financial expectations and implements production analysis using a monthly Dashboard as described in a previous publication.[14] The HIT Department performs internal data extraction, builds population registries, and has worked with Featherstone Informatics Group (FigMD) to develop an electronic interface with the American Gastroenterological Association (AGA) Digestive Health Outcomes Registry (DHOR). For details, see http://www.gastro.org/practice/digestive-health-outcomes-registry.

The cooperative philosophy of the partnership developed over the decade after the initial integration in 1998 (3 practices merged and then the practice grew by recruitment). Various compensation systems are debated, and finally (for the moment), a 50:50 split in professional income in which 50% is shared and 50% is based on production is agreed on. The shared portion is diluted by an even split of facility income from the practice-owned ambulatory surgery centers as regulated by the Stark laws, which means that only 18% of income is based on productivity, a percentage that encourages high production but narrows the margin between the highest and lowest earners. An internal quality incentive (1% of total income) is enough to focus attention on annual quality goals (mostly because of the competitive nature of the partners). As of now, there is substantial support for partners who want to develop Centers of Excellence and team-based care as long as the plans are vetted through all appropriate committees and the partnership is educated through a fair process of presentation and feedback.

HIT INFRASTRUCTURE

HIT within the practice is based on NextGen Electronic Medical Record and NextGen Enterprise Practice Management System, 2 components of a fully integrated, network-wide electronic system that records all practice functions. An internal HIT team used NextGen templates to develop an endoscopic reporting system, a pathology result reporting system (fully searchable and linked to endoscopy), registries (hepatitis C and IBD), a recall system, and templates for cognitive clinic functions (with voice recognition). The pathology database is designed using the *Systematized Nomenclature of Medicine-Clinical Terms* (SNOMED CT) terminology. Finally, the authors use the reporting functions of the electronic health record (EHR) to generate report cards and the monthly performance dashboard described previously.

The key difference between many current gastroenterology EHRs is the need for interfacing with external databases (both regional EHRs and registries), and the capabilities needed for clinical service line management include the capability of identifying specific populations, recording in a standardized (template) fashion, and implementing alerts (both proactive and retroactive). Both issues are being resolved rapidly as EHRs mature and cloud technology becomes available as a tool to integrate information from disparate data sources.

For the IBD-focused care team to succeed, standardized clinical data input should be developed and then patients who qualified for the team's care should be identified. The format suggested here is but an example of how one might construct data entry and is only partially based on what is currently present in the system. The initial screenshot of the IBD template series (for patients with Crohn's disease) is presented in **Fig. 1**.

Subsequent templates are activated for medication history and other pertinent factors. It is debated on what standard clinical points should be included in all visit dictations and firm conclusions are not yet taken, but the following items are under consideration. This means that for all new patients, the following items should appear and be repeated as often as clinically appropriate. Soon, these data elements will become menu driven and brought forward in a summary template for subsequent visits.[15]

- Pertinent demographics, family history, lifestyle data, and comorbid conditions
- Disease distribution (endoscopic, imaging, and histologic)
- Disease phenotype

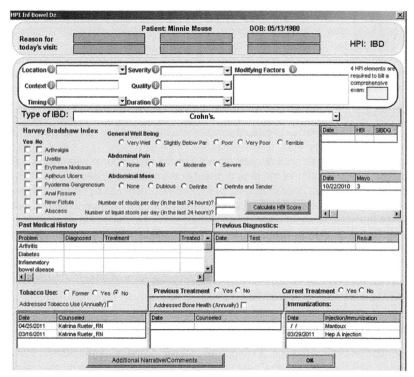

Fig. 1. The initial template for recording clinical information of patients with IBD. The template includes a disease scale (Harvey Bradshaw) and other critical information that, the authors believe, should be standard for all visits.

- Previous diagnostics with dates
- Previous surgeries
- Previous medical treatment
- Treatment complications
- Current treatment (with start dates if appropriate), especially steroid exposure
- Status of preventive measures (see below).

Identification of patients and creation of registries have presented a special challenge, but with the evolution of GI-appropriate EHRs, there will be standard terminology developed much as there was for endoscopy in the 1980s. It will be incumbent on the specialty societies to develop this common language. For now, patients are flagged using a defined set of *International Classification of Diseases, Ninth Revision* (soon to be *International Classification of Diseases, Tenth Revision*) codes used by providers when billing services. Specific registries have been built for patients on biologic therapy and immunomodulator therapy and those needing recall for laboratories, clinic visits, and endoscopic procedures (including cancer surveillance). All these registries and endoscopy and pathology databases are searchable because they were built with strict data entry definitions.

DEDICATED SPECIALISTS IN IBD

Designation of special expertise in IBD or other subspecialties of gastroenterology is usually accomplished based on personal interest and past advanced training or because a partner focuses a large portion of his or her clinical practice within a smaller subspecialized area. Within our practice, there are physicians and midlevel providers who have focused on areas such as GERD, IBD, hepatology, gastroparesis (and gastric electrical stimulation), motility, pelvic floor disorders, and each of the traditional advanced endoscopic techniques. We require evidence of ongoing educational commitment and willingness to see complex patients referred both from within the group and from external referral sources. Continuing education involves attendance at national GI meetings, review of evolving literature, involvement with the Clinical Focus Groups, presentation of patients and information at partner meetings, and other criteria as appropriate.

If a partner focuses on patients who do not generate the income seen with standard GI practice (in which 50% of the time is spent in the endoscopy center), such as IBD, functional GI disorders, hepatology, or gastroparesis, there has to be some alteration of the compensation system to recognize the importance of such work and yet still recognize the importance of revenue-generating services. Balancing competing interests requires skilled leadership and constant discussion. There is no correct answer, and discussions always evolve into negotiations. Underlying all these discussions is the willingness of the practice as a whole to support multiple facets of gastroenterology that may not currently generate the revenue of screening colonoscopy or advanced endoscopic procedures.

CLINICAL CARE ALGORITHMS AND CDS TOOLS

The foundation of any successful integrated program is the current scientific literature that helps clinicians decide the best treatments for patients. Then, further decision support tools and clinical recommendations must be made by practice experts who create triage tools for schedulers and nurses, alerts and reminders in the practice EHR, and other customized CDS tools needed for actual patient populations (as opposed to the recommendations designed from strictly defined populations within randomized controlled trials). The care pathways are based on guidelines from the AGA,[15,16] American College of Gastroenterology,[17,18] Crohn's and Colitis Foundation of America (CCFA),[19] European Crohn's and Colitis Organization,[20–22] and World Congress of Gastroenterology[23] and general health maintenance guidelines published previously.[24] The IBD Clinical Focus Group updates care pathways as newer information is published. The recommended treatment pathways are published on the practice intranet (for internal use by providers). Important concepts and studies, such as SONIC, are discussed in detail at the practice-wide meetings.[25]

Based on these guidelines and other pertinent articles, care pathways are considered to fall into 1 of 3 categories: (1) mandatory pathways that all providers within Minnesota Gastroenterology must follow, (2) strongly recommended pathways that should be followed except with that the judgment of the provider overrides the pathway for individual patients, and (3) recommended pathways but with less strength.

Examples of the first category (mandatory) include issues in which there might be liability or in which evidence is so overwhelming that deviation would be considered substandard care. Evaluating risks before prescribing certain IBD medications would be an example. Whenever a biologic therapy is ordered in the EHR, pop-up alerts appear with either recommended discussion points (cancer risk with immunomodulators) or mandated orders (tuberculosis and hepatitis B testing before biologic therapy, white blood cell counts, and a liver panel before immunomodulator therapy are examples). **Fig. 2** is the alert screen when infliximab is ordered.

Standing Orders

1. Mantoux every 2 years if the patient has had a previous negative result.
   If previous positive result, contact the provider for orders.
2. Obtain patient weight and convert to kilograms.
3. Obtain baseline set of vital signs.
4. Patient to take pre-meds at home prior to infusion.
   -If patient has not received premends, give SoluMedrol 40 mg IVx1.
   -If patient misses premeds for more than one appointment, reschedule patient and notify
      the ordering provider. Inform patient of need to take premeds at home prior to infusion.
5. If patient needs to be rescheduled on day of infliximab infusion (late for appointment, did not
   take premeds), reschedule the patient within 72 hours.
   -If an appointment time is not available within 72 hours, notify the ordering provider
      for further direction.
6. Calculate infliximab dose per physician's order (mg/kg) and divide by 100 for the number of
   infliximab vials needed
   -If the dose requires 0-25 mg of the last vial, round down.
   -If the dose requires 26-75 mg of the last vial, give the exact weight based dose and discard
      the remaining infliximab.
   -If the dose requires 76-100 mg of the last vial, round up.
7. Prime IV set with 500 mL 0.9% NS at TKO. Start IV.
8. Have available: acetaminophen 650 mg PO, SoluMedrol 40 mg IV, ranitidine 50 mg IV,
      EpiPen (epinephrine 1:1000), and diphenhydramine 50 mg IV.
9. Reconstitute Infliximab according to manufacturer's instructions, and add to 250cc 0.9% NS;
   maximum of 10 vials per 250 cc.
10. Infuse Infliximab using a 0.22/0.20 micron filter, over a minimum of 2 hours by piggyback.
11. May give acetaminophen 650 mg x1 PO for discomfort.   Titration Table
12. Monitor VS every 30 minutes, and as needed during infusion.
13. Assess patient for reaction (see reaction protocol).
14. When infusion is complete, flush Infliximab line with 20-50 mL 0.9% NS.
15. Monitor patient for 15 minutes before discharge, then discontinue IV.
16. Give patient discharge instructions.

Provider Sign Off [   ] [/ /]

These orders will be automatically signed off going forward.

Staff Sign Off: [   ] [/ /]

[OK   ]   [Cancel]

Fig. 2. The alert screen in the EHR whenever infliximab is ordered. This order set is based on the recommended procedures taken from the package insert and published guidelines[15–23] or the consensus of practice experts.

When azathioprine or 6-mercaptopurine is used, there is an automatic order set printed that defines the times when laboratory monitoring must be performed and results sent back to the practice for entry into the EHR. The system generates automatic red-flag alerts for staff if laboratory tests are not completed. Renewal of medication is delayed if patients do not comply with the orders. Patient education is designed to emphasize the importance of joint responsibility for therapy.

There is no universal agreement about many aspects of IBD care. One example would be specific timing of laboratory monitoring during immunomodulator therapy. However, the author believes that consistency at a practice level reduces the risk of liability (which is shared at a practice level). Variability among physicians within a practice, in the author's opinion, increases risk if adverse events occur.

More advanced CDS tools are needed to facilitate population management and accountability. There are examples of next-generation population-based care initiatives, some even using social media outlets. One practice in South Florida routinely identifies patients with IBD and proactively designs services and preventive care for this segment of its practice. For example, they are offered facilitated scheduling and are contacted each fall regarding the need for influenza vaccination (James Leavitt, MD, personal communication, January 2011). These initial efforts are just first steps to what needs to occur as gastroenterology takes small steps toward accountable care.[26]

One specific aspect of the care of patients with IBD in which there exits a significant gap between recommended care and care that is actually provided is in the area of preventive health services.[24] Many patients with IBD consider their gastroenterologist as their principal physician and may not have a close relationship with a PCP. This gap represents an opportunity for gastroenterologists to assume the role of PCMH-N. CDS tools are actively created to remind providers to complete recommended preventive tests whenever the opportunity exists with the patients with IBD. There is a clear need for CDS tools that integrate seamlessly within GI EHRs and care processes and should be created by pertinent national medical societies.

The feasibility of a multispecialty staffed annual preventive care visit for patients with IBD is also explored because so many such patients rely mostly (if not solely) on gastroenterologists for their medical care. Preventive health services that should be considered for patients with IBD are included in **Box 1**.[24]

Box 1
Recommended preventive services for patients with IBD

- Vaccinations
  - Tetanus, diphtheria, and pertussis
  - Human papilloma virus (for women)
  - Influenza
  - Pneumococcal
  - Hepatitis A
  - Hepatitis B
  - Meningococcal
  - Measles, mumps, and rubella
  - Varicella (live vaccine)
  - Herpes zoster (live vaccine)
- Laboratory monitoring before initiation of therapy and during therapy
  - Tuberculosis and viral hepatitis assessment
  - Complete blood count, liver function testing, creatinine, C-reactive protein, and sedimentation rate as appropriate during medication therapy
  - B-12 and folic acid testing or replacement
  - Vitamin D
- Tobacco cessation

Data from Moscandrew M, Mahadevan U, Kane S. General health maintenance in IBD. Inflamm Bowel Dis 2009;15:1399–408.

OUTCOME MEASURES

Although CDS tools are designed to give direction to providers in a dynamic, point-of-care manner, outcome measures are needed to look back at how successful providers are at improving medical outcomes and providing health value to patients, both individually and at a population level. Measures are created to help patients, providers, payers, and purchasers know that the care given to people is safe, timely, effective, efficient, equitable, and patient centered. These are the 6 aims of the Institute of Medicine reports on quality in American health care, published more than a decade ago.[27] Recently, a review of quality measures that is specific for gastroenterology conditions has been published.[28] The process of creating, validating, endorsing, and implementing performance improvement and accountability measures in the United States is now organized and follows a clear pathway.[29] If outcomes measures are to be used for incentive payments or even as internal accountability measures, they should reflect important patient outcomes and be endorsed by a national recognized entity such as the National Quality Forum. Over the past 2 years, a joint task force of the AGA and CCFA (in cooperation with other groups) has produced a set of measures related to IBD.[30] Current IBD measures are listed in **Box 2**. These measures are now incorporated into the DHOR, which was developed by the AGA to encompass a wide range of gastroenterology outcome measures. The IBD measures have been now endorsed by the Centers for Medicare and Medicaid for use in the 2012 Physician Quality Reporting System and represent a validated and endorsed set of measures that can be used by a practice, health care system, or health plan to evaluate IBD care at a provider or practice level. As part of a comprehensive IBD Center of Excellence, performance measurement has become important to demonstrate practice commitment to quality improvement and accountable care.

Box 2
Adult IBD physician performance measure set. Ten outcome measures submitted to CMS and NQF by a joint task force from the AGA and CCFA. At present, eight outpatient measures have been accepted into PQRS and will likely appear in 2012. They will be submitted to NQF in 2012 during their call for measures

Measure 1. IBD type, anatomic location, and activity all assessed

Measure 2. IBD preventive care: corticosteroid sparing therapy

Measure 3. IBD preventive care: corticosteroid-related iatrogenic injury—bone loss assessment

Measure 4. IBD preventive care: influenza immunization

Measure 5. IBD preventive care: pneumococcal immunization

Measure 6. Screening for latent tuberculosis before initiating anti–tumor necrosis factor (TNF) therapy

Measure 7. Assessment of hepatitis B virus before initiating anti-TNF therapy

Measure 8. Testing for *Clostridium difficile*—inpatient measure

Measure 9. Prophylaxis for venous thromboembolism—inpatient measure

Measure 10. IBD preventive care: tobacco user—screening and cessation intervention

Abbreviations: AGA, American Gastroenterological Association; CCFA, Crohn's and Colitis Foundation of America; CMS, Centers for Medicare and Medicaid; NQF, National Quality Forum; PQRS, Physician Quality and Reporting System.

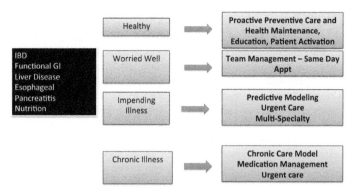

Fig. 3. Restructuring practice to include chronic care model. For patients with chronic conditions (see the list on left), there are 4 major categories (middle column). Each of these types of patients needs a slightly different practice infrastructure to rapidly meet their needs. Examples of the needed infrastructure are illustrated in the right-hand column.

FINANCIAL ANALYSIS AND DEVELOPMENT OF TREATMENT TEAMS

The last steps a practice can take to develop a PCMH-N for IBD is the development of sophisticated financial analysis of resource use and Lean analysis.[12] Within advanced EHRs and practice management systems resides the capability of creating performance dashboards and resource analysis. For now, it is a difficult task to assign responsibility for resource use by a single patient to specific providers. For example, which resource use is assigned to PCP versus specialist in the treatment of patients with multiple medical conditions? Most large group practices cross-cover partners' patients so that a single individual might not be responsible for all resource use for a specific patient. Within an integrated health care system, such analysis is more defined, but such is not the case when multiple independent specialty groups are associated with a hospital system and PCPs. There is a rapid evolution of Episode Grouper Methodology[31] and attribution models; hence, payments and accountability based on episode of care will emerge within the next few years. Within a group looking to establish population management of a group of patients with IBD, it is not as important to analyze to the provider level. A practice should be able to define resources they (the practice) used in the care of a defined set of patients. Internal analysis of practice trends and emphasis on evidence-based decisions both would be important to transitioning to bundled payments and episode-based analysis.

A team-based approach has been successfully used in the diagnosis and care of some groups of patients, such as those with complex esophageal disease and chronic liver disease. Patients are educated about the team and can access multiple providers who are familiar with their situation. This will be extending this to IBD as the program matures. The most important aspect of IBD team-based care will be the ability to respond in different ways to the differing needs of patients. **Fig. 3** illustrates the 4 basic types of patients with chronic conditions.

SUMMARY

Changing practices from a reactive consultant model to a proactive population management approach is difficult but will allow practices to evolve into an infrastructure that will be attractive to patients and health care systems. It is believed that building a practice model such as the one illustrated in this article will allow us, as a large independent gastroenterology practice, to offer the highest value service while remaining independent and affiliated with multiple ACOs or hospital systems. Needed advances are awaited in EHRs, information management, CDS tools, additional guidelines, and outcomes measurement to more fully implement this practice model.

REFERENCES

1. Shortell SM, Casalino LP. Health care reform requires accountable care systems. JAMA 2008;300:95–7.
2. Fisher ES, Shortell SM. Accountable care organizations: accountable for what, to whom and how. JAMA 2010;304:1715–6.
3. Enthoven AC. Reforming Medicare by reforming incentives. N Engl J Med 2011; 364:1887–90.
4. Jain SH, Cassel CK. Societal perceptions of physicians—knights, knaves or pawns? JAMA 2010;304:1009–10.
5. Kocher R, Sahni NR. Physicians versus hospitals as leaders of accountable care organizations. N Engl J Med 2010;363:2579–82.
6. Berwick DM, Nolan TW, Whittington J. The triple aim: care, health and cost. Health Aff (Millwood) 2008;27:759–69.
7. Bodenheimer T. Lessons from the trenches—a high-functioning primary care clinic. N Engl J Med 2011;365:5–8.
8. Porter ME, Teisberg EO. How physicians can change the future of health care. JAMA 2007;297:1103–11.
9. Kirschner N, Greenlee MC. The patient-centered medical home neighbor: the interface of the patient-centered medical home with specialty/subspecialty practices. A position paper of the American College of Physicians. 2010. Available at: www.acponline.org/fcgi/search?q=patient+centered+medical+neighborhood&;site= ACP_Online&x=0&y=0. Accessed August 6, 2011.
10. Reschovsky JD, Hadley J, Saiontz-Martinez S, et al. Following the money: factors associated with the cost of treating high-cost Medicare beneficiaries. Health Serv Res 2011;46:997–1021.
11. Kocher R, Sahni NR. Hospital's race to employ physicians—the logic behind a money-losing proposition. N Engl J Med 2011;364:1790–3.
12. Murphree P, Vath RR, Daigle L. Sustaining lean six sigma projects in health care. Physician Exec 2011;37:44–8.
13. Schechter MS, Margolis P. Improving subspecialty healthcare: lessons from cystic fibrosis. J Pediatr 2005;147:295–301.
14. Allen JI. A performance improvement program for community-based gastroenterology. Gastrointest Endosc Clin N Am 2008;18:753–71.
15. Lichtenstein GR, Abreu MT, Cohen R, et al. American Gastroenterology Association Institute medical position statement on corticosteroids, immunomodulators, and infliximab in inflammatory bowel disease. Gastroenterology 2006;130:935–9.
16. Farraye FA, Odze RD, Eaden J, et al. AGA medical position statement on the diagnosis and management of colorectal neoplasia in inflammatory bowel disease. Gastroenterology 2010;138:738–45.
17. Lichtenstein GR, Hanauer SB, Sandborn WJ, et al. Management of Crohn's disease in adults. Am J Gastroenterol 2009;104:465–83.
18. Kornbluth A, Sachar DB, Practice Parameters Committee of the American College of Gastroenterology. Ulcerative colitis practice guidelines in adults: American College of Gastroenterology, Practice Parameters Committee. Am J Gastroenterol 2010;105:501–23.

19. Itzkowitz SH, Present DH, Crohn's and Colitis Foundation of America Colon Cancer in IBD Study Group. Consensus conference: colorectal cancer screening and surveillance in inflammatory bowel disease. Inflamm Bowel Dis 2005;11: 314–21.

20. Dignass A, Van Assche G, Lindsay JO, et al. The second European evidence-based consensus on the diagnosis and management of Crohn's disease: current management. J Crohns Colitis 2010;4:28–62.

21. Van Assche G, Dignass A, Panes J, et al. The second European evidence-based consensus on the diagnosis and management of Crohhn's disease: definitions and diagnosis. J Crohns Colitis 2010;4:7–27.

22. Van Assche G, Dignass A, Reinisch W, et al. The second European evidence-based consensus on the diagnosis and management of Crohn's disease: special situations. J Crohns Colitis 2010;4:63–101.

23. Bernstein CN, Fried M, Krabshuis JH, et al. World Gastroenterology Organisation Practice Guideline—inflammatory bowel disease: a global perspective. Available at: http://www.worldgastroenterology.org/inflammatory-bowel-disease.html. Accessed August 10, 2011.

24. Moscandrew M, Mahadevan U, Kane S. General health maintenance in IBD. Inflamm Bowel Dis 2009;15:1399–408.

25. Colombei JF, Sandborn WJ, Reinisch W, et al. Infliximab, azathioprine, or combination therapy for Crohn's disease. N Engl J Med 2010;362:1383–95.

26. Allen JI. Baby epsilon steps towards the Triple Aim. Gastroenterology 2011;140: 1129–31.

27. Institute of Medicine. Crossing the quality chasm: a new health system for the 21st century. Washington, DC: National Academy Press; 2001.

28. Kappelman MD, Dorn SD, Peterson E, et al. Quality of care for gastrointestinal conditions: a primer for gastroenterologists. Am J Gastroenterol 2011;106: 1182–7.

29. Corrigan JM, Burstin H. Measuring quality of performance: where is it headed, and who is making the decisions? J Fam Pract 2007;56:4a–7a.

30. Executive Managment Board of the Registry and the Governing Board of AGA Institute. Available at: http://www.gastro.org/practice/digestive-health-outcomes-registry/clinical-content/ibd-measures. Accessed August 11, 2011.

31. Forthman MT, Dove HG, Wooster LD. Episode treatment groups (ETGs): a patient classification system for measuring outcomes performance by episode of illness. Top Health Inf Manage 2000;21(2):51–61.

The Impact of Health Reform on Gastroenterology Reimbursement

Joel V. Brill, MD

KEYWORDS

- Reimbursement • Health care costs • Affordable Care Act
- Health reform

Unless one has been living on a desert island without newspapers, cellular service, or access to the Internet for the past few years, one would understand that the rising costs of health care and its impact on the current and future economic status of the United States have been a significant factor in guiding our domestic policy agenda. During the 2008 Presidential campaign, the candidates were challenged to articulate their proposals for health reform in the middle of the worst economic recession since the Great Depression.

The candidates' approach to addressing an environment where many working families were without medical insurance or had burdensome medical expenses could not have been more different. Over the decade, cumulative increases in health insurance premiums were more than 130%, greatly outstripping a 38% increase in workers' earnings that was offset by a 28% increase in inflation.[1,2] While both candidates proposed plans to reform the health insurance system while improving the quality and efficiency of care, Obama's proposal for private-public group insurance with a shared responsibility for financing significantly differed from McCain's proposal to encourage individual market coverage through the use of tax incentives and deregulation.[3] The fundamental differences between the Republican and Democratic proposals are summarized in **Table 1**.

One problem with our current payment system is that physicians, hospitals, and other health care providers are financially incented to deliver more services to more

Disclosures: There is no discussion of unapproved or use of off-label products. Board of Directors: American Board of Quality Assurance and Utilization Review Physicians, Inc, AGA Digestive Health Outcomes Registry, Early Bird Alert, Inc, Endochoice. Personal Possession of Shares/Options: Early Bird Alert, Endochoice, Given Imaging. Consulting: Avantis Medical, Barrx Medical, Exalenz Bioscience, Given Imaging, Salix Pharmaceuticals, The Smart Pill Corporation.
Predictive Health, LLC, 6245 North 24th Parkway, Suite 112, Phoenix, AZ 85016, USA
E-mail address: joel.brill@gmail.com

Gastrointest Endoscopy Clin N Am 22 (2012) 97–107
doi:10.1016/j.giec.2011.08.001   giendo.theclinics.com
1052-5157/12/$ – see front matter © 2012 Elsevier Inc. All rights reserved.

Table 1 Republican and Democratic health insurance proposals		
	Republican	Democrat
Aim to cover everybody	Not a goal	Goal
Employer role in providing health benefits	Reduce	Expand
Medicaid	Reduce	Expand
Families' exposure to health care costs	More	Less
Stimulate improvement in quality and efficiency	No change	More

people (volume-driven), but that the payment systems do not recognize efforts to improve health (value-driven). Current systems which assume that all providers have equivalent quality fail to encourage the use of high-value providers.[4] Our fee-for-service payment system is not designed to bundle the services of different providers into a single-episode payment, even if all of those services are integral parts of a patient's total episode of care. Thus, most discussions about health care payment reform have focused on methods for paying providers—medical homes, episode-based payment, and comprehensive care payments—whose goal is to avoid providing unnecessary services within any particular episode of care.[5] An episode payment is a single price for all of the services needed by a patient for an entire episode of care (eg, colorectal cancer screening). Comprehensive care payment, also referred to as risk-adjusted global fees or condition-adjusted capitation, is a population-based approach whereby a single price is paid for all of the health care services needed by a specific group of people for a fixed period of time.[6] While there are advantages and disadvantages to different payment methods and incentives, one must keep in mind that if the payment level is below the cost of providing care, providers will be unable to provide quality care.[7]

Along with concerns about costs has been a focus on patient value. While the goals may be to improve the quality, safety, efficiency, and value of care, the current focus has been on pay-for-performance, value-driven health care, and public reporting of quality and cost information. Pay-for-performance programs from Medicare, Medicaid, and commercial payors have been uncoordinated, and process reporting may not be clearly aligned with producing better outcomes for patients.[8,9] Although steps have been taken to align quality and value efforts with improving care for patients, payment for high-quality, efficient care that rewards achievement of improved patient outcomes over episodes of care while minimizing the opportunity for unintended negative consequences requires reform of payment methodologies.[10]

The Patient Protection and Affordable Care Act (Public Law 111-148) was signed into law on March 23, 2010. Following the enactment of Public Law 111-148, the Health Care and Education Reconciliation Act of 2010 (Public Law 111-152) (enacted on March 30, 2010), amended certain provisions of Public Law 111-148. These public laws are collectively known as the Affordable Care Act. The Affordable Care Act includes several provisions designed to improve the quality of Medicare services, support innovation and the establishment of new payment models in the program, better align Medicare payments with provider costs, strengthen program integrity within Medicare, and put Medicare on a firmer financial footing.

There are several provisions in the Affordable Care Act that will affect gastroenterology. Section 3022 of the Affordable Care Act amended Title XVIII of the Social Security Act (the Act) (42 U.S.C. 1395 et seq.) by adding new section 1899 to the Act to establish a Shared Savings Program that promotes accountability for a patient population, coordinates items and services under Parts A and B, and encourages investment in infrastructure and redesigned care processes for high-quality and efficient service delivery. Section 1899(a)(1) of the Act requires the Secretary of the Department of Health and Human Services (HHS) to establish this program no later than January 1, 2012. Section 1899(a)(1)(A) of the Act further provides that "groups of providers of services and suppliers meeting criteria specified by the Secretary may work together to manage and coordinate care for Medicare fee-for-service beneficiaries through an [ACO]" (Accountable Care Organization). Section 1899(a)(1)(B) of the Act also provides that ACOs that meet quality performance standards established by the Secretary are eligible to receive payments for "shared savings." On March 31, 2011 the Centers for Medicare and Medicaid Services (CMS) released a notice of proposed rulemaking for the Medicare Shared Savings Program, which would allow eligible providers, hospitals, and suppliers to voluntarily participate in the Shared Savings Program by creating or joining an ACO.[11] While the proposed rule allowed specialists to participate in multiple ACOs, whether organized by primary care physicians and/or hospitals, the rule did not allow specialists to organize ACOs.

One might anticipate that while specialists will initially be paid under a fee-for-service methodology in an ACO, payment could transition to a methodology around episodes of care such as colorectal cancer screening, viral hepatitis, inflammatory bowel disease, esophageal disorders, metabolic disorders, and malnutrition. Payment could be based on a formula combining fee-for-service payments and achieving definable outcomes, such as the percentage of the population receiving colorectal cancer screening and the physician's adherence to multispecialty consensus guidelines around intervals for follow-up surveillance. When the ACO is financially responsible for the health of a population, the question is not whether the all-in price of the colonoscopy (endoscopist, facility, pathology, sedation, pharmaceuticals, and complications) is $1000 or $5000; it is whether the service needs to be purchased at all. Thus, one question for gastroenterologists is whether they wish to be at the end of the food chain dependent on referrals for screening colonoscopy, or whether they wish to advance to the head of the food chain by assuming responsibility for the rate of colorectal cancer screening in the population served, choosing to deploy the variety of noninvasive and invasive screening methods based on the individualized need by each patient.

The current Medicare payment system includes one payment for the facility and one payment for the physician. Because payment is unique to each site of service, providers do not have financial incentives to provide care that will reduce costs in other locations. Bundling refers to the policy of linking payment for services to an entire episode of care. Section 3023 as amended by Section 10308 requires the Secretary to develop, test, and evaluate Medicare payment methodologies through a voluntary pilot program for integrated care to improve the coordination, quality, and efficiency of health care services. This "bundled payment" program requires the establishment of a national pilot program on payment bundling for the Medicare program by January 1, 2013 and a Medicaid bundling demonstration program by 2012, and may be expanded after January 1, 2016 if the Secretary determines that expansion would reduce spending without reducing the quality of care, and would not deny or limit coverage or provision of benefits for beneficiaries. In conducting the pilot program, the Secretary will test alternative payment methods, which may include bundled payments and include payment for services such as care coordination, medication reconciliation, discharge planning, transitional care services, and other patient-centered activities. The demonstration sets the episode of care to begin

3 days before the hospital admission and end 30 days following hospital discharge. Bundled payments would cover the costs of acute-care inpatient services, physician services delivered in and outside of an acute-care hospital setting, outpatient hospital services including emergency department services, and post–acute-care services.[12] One could foresee where this proposal could affect payment when a patient suffers a complication, such as a perforation or bleeding after an index endoscopic procedure.

Section 3002 of the Act describes improvements to the Physician Quality Reporting System (PQRS), as modified by Section 10327. Eligible professionals (EP) who successfully report quality data will receive a 1.0% bonus in 2011 and a 0.5% bonus in years 2012 through 2014. EPs who do not successfully report quality data will have their Medicare payments reduced by 1.5% in 2015 and 2.0% in 2016 and each subsequent year. The payment incentives and reductions are based on the Medicare fee schedule amounts for all covered services furnished by the EP. This section also increases the PQRS incentive payment by 0.5% for years 2011 to 2014 for EPs for whom required quality data is submitted for a year on their behalf by a qualified American Board of Medical Specialists Maintenance of Certification (MOC) or equivalent program that meets the criteria for a registry; and which, more frequently than is required for board certification, participate in a MOC and complete a qualified MOC practice assessment. For years after 2014, the Secretary can incorporate participation in an MOC program and successful completion of a qualified MOC program practice assessment into the composite of measures of quality of care for the purposes of the physician fee schedule value-based payment modifier, as outlined in Section 3007.

Sections 3001 (Hospital Value-Based Purchasing Program), 3004 (Quality Reporting Requirements for Long-Term Care Hospitals, Inpatient Rehabilitation Hospitals, Inpatient Psychiatric Hospitals and Hospice Program), 3006 (Skilled Nursing Facility, Home Health Agency and Ambulatory Surgical Center Value-Based Purchasing Program), 3007 (Value-Based Payment Modifier Under the Medicare Physician Fee Schedule), 10322 (Availability of Medicare Data for Performance Measurement), and 10326 (Medicare Pay-For-Performance Pilot Program) of the Act advance several new payment and delivery system proposals to promote value-based purchasing in the Medicare program.[13] On January 7, 2011, CMS released a proposed rule to implement a hospital value-based purchasing program, which would apply to payments for discharges occurring on or after October 1, 2012, and would reward with higher payments hospitals that score well on quality care measures. The proposal includes quality measures around surgical care activities, health care–associated infections, and patient perceptions of care.[14]

Section 3007, the Value-Based Purchasing Modifier, provides for the Secretary to implement a budget-neutral payment system that adjusts the Medicare physician fee schedule based on the quality and cost of the care delivered, including geographically standardized risk adjustments for quality and cost measures. The system will be phased in over a 2-year period beginning January 1, 2015. The modifier is separate from and does not replace the geographic adjustment factors, and should promote systems-based care. The Secretary is directed to establish a composite of appropriate risk-based measures of quality, which must be submitted to the National Quality Forum for endorsement. In addition, the Secretary will establish a composite of appropriate measures of costs.

By 2017, episode-based cost measures developed using the public Medicare-specific episode grouper software also may be considered in developing a composite score. An "episode grouper" is software that organizes claims data into clinically coherent episodes of care across different providers, which includes all contacts with the health care system for a specific health problem between a start and end point, and will allow CMS to compare risk-adjusted costs of care for similar patients across physicians. Section 1848(n)(9)(A) of the Act, as added by Section 3003 of the Affordable Care Act, requires the development, by not later than January 1, 2012, of a Medicare-specific episode grouper so that physicians can be compared on episode-based costs of care. The episode grouper will require further testing and refinement to see how well it integrates with other parameters, such as attribution and benchmarking, before it can be fully operational. The episode grouper is being developed to determine episode-based costs for a subset of selected high-cost, high-volume conditions for Medicare beneficiaries.

On July 1, 2011, CMS released the Medicare Physician Fee Schedule Proposed Rule for CY 2012, where they identified proposed quality of care measures for the Value-Based Modifier.[15] For purposes of Section 1848(p)(4)(A)(i) of the Act, CMS proposes to use performance on: (1) the measures in the core set of the PQRS for 2012; (2) all measures in the Group Practice Reporting Option (GPRO) of the Physician Quality Reporting System for 2012; and (3) the core measures, alternate core, and 38 additional measures in the Electronic Health Record Incentive Program measures for 2012. While CMS has requested input on quality measures that assess the care provided by specialists, the proposal includes several measures that could be reported by gastroenterologists, including:

- 110: Influenza immunization
- 111: Pneumococcal vaccination
- 113: Colorectal cancer screening
- 128: Body mass index screening and follow-up
- 239: Weight assessment and counseling for children and adolescents
- 226: Tobacco use screening and cessation intervention
- 237: Blood pressure measurement
- TBD: Proportion of patients (18+) who have had their blood pressure measured in the past 2 years
- 46: Medication reconciliation after discharge from inpatient facility.

Section 3006(f) of the Act, as added by Section 10301(a), requires the Secretary to develop a plan to implement a value-based purchasing (VBP) program for payments under the Medicare program for ambulatory surgical centers (ASCs). Gastroenterology is the top Specialty category by volume for ASC claims, constituting 32.7% of claims in CY 2009, and endoscopic procedures (esophagogastroduodenoscopy [EGD] with biopsy, colonoscopy with biopsy, diagnostic colonoscopy) constitute 3 of the top 5 surgical procedures by volume.[16] In the proposed rule that would update the hospital Outpatient Prospective Payment System (OPPS) and ASC payment system for 2012, CMS is now proposing to implement a quality reporting system under which data collection would begin in 2012.[17] For the first 2 years, ASCs would not be financially penalized for failure to report quality information. However, beginning in 2014, CMS would begin reducing Medicare payments to ASCs that fail to report data on specified quality measures. For 2015, CMS has proposed to collect ASC volume data on selected ASC procedures. Both surgeon volume and facility volume are correlated with surgical outcomes and that higher volumes correspond to better performance. These data and analyses are specific to discrete surgical procedures. For the ASC procedure volume measure, CMS proposes collecting and reporting surgical volume not for specific procedures, but across a range of procedure codes that will be aggregated and reported by broad categories. It is not clear, however, that the same statistical relationships exist when procedure-specific data are aggregated into much broader categories. CMS is soliciting comments on the inclusion of procedure-specific measures for colonoscopy and endoscopy, and for measures of anesthesia-related complications.

The most significant challenge to gastroenterology is the question of whether physician payments are appropriate. Medicare pays for physician services based on a list of services and their payment rates, called the physician fee schedule. In determining payment rates for each service on the fee schedule, CMS considers the amount of work required to provide a service, expenses related to maintaining a practice, and liability insurance costs. The values given to these 3 types of resources are adjusted by variations in the input prices in different markets, then a total is multiplied by a standard dollar amount, called the fee schedule's conversion factor, to arrive at the payment amount. Medicare's payment rates may be adjusted based on provider characteristics, additional geographic designations, and other factors. The conversion factor updates payments for physician services every year according to a formula called the sustainable growth rate (SGR) system. This formula is intended to keep spending growth (a function of service volume growth) consistent with growth in the national economy. However, in the last several years, Congress has specified an update outside of the SGR formula.

Under the fee schedule payment system, payment rates are based on relative weights, called relative value units (RVUs), which account for the relative costliness of the inputs used to provide physician services: physician work, practice expenses, and professional liability insurance (PLI) expenses. The RVUs for physician work reflect the relative levels of time, effort, skill, and stress associated with providing each service. The RVUs for practice expense are based on the expenses physicians incur when they rent office space, buy supplies and equipment, and hire nonphysician clinical and administrative staff. The PLI RVUs are based on the premiums physicians pay for professional liability/medical malpractice insurance.

In calculating payment rates, each of the 3 RVUs is adjusted to reflect the price level for related inputs in the local market where the service is furnished. Separate geographic practice cost indexes (GPCIs) are used for this purpose. The fee schedule payment amount is then determined by summing the adjusted weights and multiplying the total by the fee schedule conversion factor. For most physician services, Medicare pays the provider 80% of the fee schedule amount. The beneficiary is liable for the remaining 20% coinsurance.[18]

In the CY 2011 Physician Fee Schedule proposed rule, CMS solicited public comments on possible approaches and methodologies for a validation process.[19] As discussed in the CY 2011 Physician Fee Schedule final rule, several commentators were skeptical that there could be viable alternative methods to the existing American Medical Association's (AMA) Relative Value Update Committee (RUC) code review process for validating physician time and intensity that would preserve the appropriate relativity of specific physician's services under the current payment system, urging CMS to rely solely on the RUC to provide valuations for services.[20] However, others expressed support for the development and establishment of a system-wide validation process of the work RVUs. Other alternatives included the use of time and motion studies to validate estimates of physician time and intensity, and the Medicare Payment Advisory Committee (MedPAC) suggested "collecting data on a recurring basis from a cohort of practices and other facilities where physicians and nonphysician clinical practitioners work."[21]

Section 3134 of the Affordable Care Act requires the Secretary to periodically review and identify potentially misvalued codes and make appropriate adjustments to their relative values, including services that have experienced high growth rates. Section

3134(a) of the Affordable Care Act added a new section, 1848(c)(2)(K) of the Act, that requires the Secretary to periodically identify potentially misvalued services using certain criteria, and to review and make appropriate adjustments to the relative values for those services. Section 3134(a) of the Affordable Care Act also added a new section, 1848(c)(2)(L) of the Act, which requires the Secretary to develop a validation process to validate the RVUs of certain potentially misvalued codes under the physician fee schedule, identified using the same categorical criteria used to identify potentially misvalued codes, and to make appropriate adjustments. The validation process may include validation of work elements (such as time, mental effort and professional judgment, technical skill and physical effort, and stress due to risk) involved with furnishing a service and may include validation of the preservice, postservice, and intraservice components of work. The Secretary is directed to validate a sampling of the work RVUs of codes identified through any of the 7 categories of potentially misvalued codes specified by Section 1848(c)(2)(K)(ii) of the Act. In the Physician Fee Schedule proposed rule for 2012, CMS proposes "to consolidate the formal Five-Year Review of Work and PE [practice expense] with the annual review of potentially misvalued codes." CMS would begin meeting the statutory requirement to review work and PE RVUs for potentially misvalued codes at least once every 5 years through an annual process, rather than once every 5 years. Furthermore, CMS has proposed a process by which the public could submit codes for potential review, which would be incorporated into their potentially misvalued codes initiative. The validation process may include validation of work elements (such as time, mental effort and professional judgment, technical skill and physical effort, and stress due to risk) involved with furnishing a service and may include validation of the pre-, post-, and intraservice components of work.

CMS emphasizes the need to review codes that are identified as part of the potentially misvalued initiative to ensure that appropriate relativity is constructed and maintained in several key relationships: that work and PE RVUs of codes are ranked appropriately within the code family; that work and PE RVUs of codes are appropriately relative based on comparison of physician time and/or intensity and/or direct inputs to other services furnished by physicians in the same specialty; and that work and PE RVUs of codes are appropriately relative when compared with services across specialties. What this means for gastroenterology is that all of our endoscopy codes could be targeted for review between now and 2013. CMS will look at the procedure times to ensure that relativity is appropriately constructed and maintained within a family of codes. This review may bring to the forefront the question of whether there is a difference in procedure time between those who administer their own sedation for average-risk patients undergoing endoscopic procedures and those who use sedation administered by an anesthesia professional.

Several codes that affect gastroenterology have already been identified by CMS for review by the RUC. In the CY 2011 Physician Fee Schedule final rule, CMS requested that the societies survey codes 43239 (EGD/biopsy), 45330 (flexible sigmoidoscopy), 45380 (colonoscopy/biopsy), and 45385 (colonoscopy/polypectomy). As a result of the fastest growing services screen, in May 2011 the RUC asked the gastrointestinal societies to explain the growth in services of codes 43259 (EGD with endoscopic ultrasound [EUS]), 43242 (EGD, EUS with fine-needle aspiration), 43236 (EGD with injection), and 45381 (colonoscopy with injection). In the Five-Year Review of Work Relative Value Units Under the Physician Fee Schedule published on June 6, 2011, CMS asks for a review of the ERCP (endoscopic retrograde cholangiopancreatography) code family.[22] In the Physician Fee Schedule proposed rule for 2012, CMS asks the societies to review the physician work and practice expense of codes

43235 (EGD), 45378 (colonoscopy), 96413 (chemotherapy administration, intravenous infusion, up to 1 hour), and 88305 (Level IV—surgical pathology, gross and microscopic examination), noting that because these codes have significant impact on physician fee schedule payment on a specialty level, a review of the relativity of the code to ensure that the work and PE RVUs are appropriately relative within the specialty and across specialties is essential.

In the proposed rule for 2012, CMS has also requested that the RUC conduct a comprehensive review of all evaluation and management (E/M) codes. Noting the significant interest in delivery system reform, such as patient-centered medical homes and making the primary care physician the focus of managing the patient's chronic conditions, CMS believes the focus of primary care has evolved from an episodic treatment–based orientation to a focus on comprehensive patient-centered care management to meet the challenges of preventing and managing chronic disease.

Section 3403(b) of the Affordable Care Act establishes an Independent Payment Advisory Board (IPAB) "to extend Medicare solvency and reduce spending growth through the use of a spending target system and fast-track legislative approval process." This Board must submit recommendations to Congress, beginning in 2014, to reduce the growth of Medicare expenditures while maintaining or improving the quality of care delivered. The Board is to be composed of 15 members appointed by the President with the advice and consent of the Senate. By April 30 of each year—beginning in 2013—the CMS Office of the Actuary will project whether Medicare's per-capita spending growth rate in the following 2 years will exceed a targeted rate. If future Medicare spending is expected to exceed the targets, the IPAB will propose recommendations to Congress and the President to reduce the growth rate. The IPAB's first set of recommendations would be proposed on January 15, 2014 and would be implemented on January 1, 2015. If Congress fails to pass legislation by August 15 of each year to achieve the required savings through other policy changes, the IPAB's recommendations will automatically take effect. Hospitals and hospices will not be subject to cost reductions proposed by the IPAB from 2015 through 2019. Beginning July 1, 2014, the IPAB must also submit an annual report providing information on system-wide health care costs; patient access to care; utilization; and quality of care that allows comparison by region, types of services, types of providers, and payers—both private insurers and Medicare. It is clear that to achieve the required savings, the obvious option will be for the IPAB to make recommendations that would decrease physician payments.

Section 6301 of the Affordable Care Act amends the Social Security Act (42 USC 1301et seq.) to add a new Part D on comparative clinical effectiveness research. Comparative clinical effectiveness research means research that evaluates and compares the patient health outcomes and benefits of 2 or more medical treatments or services. Such treatment and services are defined broadly to include protocols for treatment, care management, and delivery; procedures; diagnostic tools; medical devices; therapeutics; and any other strategies used to treat, diagnose, or prevent illness or injury. This process establishes the Patient-Centered Outcomes Research Institute (PCORI), responsible for the identification, prioritization, and execution of such comparative effectiveness research. The PCORI is structured as a tax-exempt independent government corporation overseen by a board of governors, responsible for setting national clinical comparative effectiveness research priorities and directed to enter into contracts to manage the funding and conduct of research. The PCORI will be responsible for establishing a standing research methodologies committee to develop standards for clinical comparative effectiveness, but the PCORI will conduct no research itself. The PCORI is required to appoint advisory panels that are expert in performing randomized clinical trials under the PCORI's research project agenda, and to appoint an expert advisory panel for purposes of assisting in the design of research studies and in determining the value and feasibility of conducting research studies for rare diseases. Measures will be developed to assess quality through comparative effectiveness, but also to assess value, which will likely include an evaluation of comparative cost and patient compliance factors, such as treatment regimen and unpleasant or harmful side effects. Research will be funded by the newly established Patient-Centered Outcomes Research Trust Fund (PCORTF), which will receive appropriations from private insurance–based taxes. PCORI offers an opportunity for physicians and medical device manufacturers to demonstrate the benefits of their interventions in specific subpopulations, which may lead to coverage and reimbursement.

Section 3021 creates a Center for Medicare and Medicaid Innovation to test payment and service delivery models that reduce costs while preserving or enhancing the quality of care. The Secretary may limit model testing to certain geographic areas, and model designs do not initially have to ensure budget neutrality. The Innovation Center "evaluate[s] each model on the quality of care furnished and the changes in spending," and its mandate provides great flexibility in selecting and testing innovative payment and service delivery models. It also allows the Secretary to expand, through rule making, the scope and duration of models proven effective after evaluation, including implementation on a nationwide basis. To expand a model, the Secretary must determine that the model improves the quality of patient care, and the CMS Actuary must certify that expanding the program will lower costs (or at least not increase costs).

One of the Innovation Center's initial proposals is the Pioneer ACO Model, which is designed for health care organizations and providers that are already experienced in coordinating care for patients across care settings. This model will allow these provider groups to move more rapidly from a shared savings payment model to a population-based payment model on a track consistent with, but separate from, the Medicare Shared Savings Program. It is designed to work in coordination with private payers by aligning provider incentives, which will improve quality and health outcomes for patients across the ACO, and achieve cost savings for Medicare, employers, and patients. The payment models being tested in the first 2 years of the Pioneer ACO Model are a shared savings payment policy with generally higher levels of shared savings and risk for Pioneer ACOs than levels currently proposed in the Medicare Shared Savings Program. In year 3 of the program, participating ACOs that have shown a specified level of savings over the first 2 years will be eligible to move a substantial portion of their payments to a population-based model.

In this era of challenges to reimbursement and change, what is a gastroenterologist to do? First is to recognize that one's success will depend on creating a system of learning through practice redesign that incorporates systems engineering tools, team-based care, and electronic medical record functionality. Leadership, governance, and culture-aligned incentives are critical, because those who have figured out how to manage internal variation will come out ahead. Second is to take a critical look at how one's practice operates. Are you operating in an efficient manner? Have you looked critically at "who does what" to maximize your margins? Have you assessed your referral sources to determine which ones are likely to be bought by a hospital or medical group? Have you reviewed your referrals to see who your top payors are by referring physicians, the contribution of each payor to gross revenues, and the impact if there is a shift in referral sources? Third is to recognize that we are moving toward a gastroenterology outcomes set whereby we will be measured on how our efforts improve the patient's experience of care, encouraging better health for populations while reducing costs. We will be measured on our colorectal cancer screening rates and surveillance intervals, adherence with preventive measures, improvement in patient safety, reduction in infections and other complications, and compliance with evidence-based care for gastrointestinal conditions including hepatitis, inflammatory bowel disease, obesity, gastroesophageal reflux disease, and dyspepsia. The National Quality Forum has already considered, and declined to endorse, quality measures based solely on documentation of endoscopic procedures. Fourth, gastroenterologists should consider that what worked in the past might not necessarily be the formula for success in this decade. In an era of comprehensive care payments, collaboration—not competition—may be the mantra for success. Gastroenterologists should be prepared to measure and report on what they do, and remain open to exploring how joint ventures with hospitals and risk-bearing medical groups may position them to thrive, not just survive, in the future.

REFERENCES

1. Kaiser Family Foundation, Health Research and Education Trust. Kaiser/HRET survey of employer health benefits. Menlo Park (CA): KFF; 2010.
2. Claxton G, DiJulio B, Whitmore H, et al. Health benefits in 2010: premiums rise modestly, workers pay more toward coverage. Health Aff (Millwood) 2010; 29(10):1942–50.
3. Collins SR, Nicholson JL, Rustgi SD, et al. The 2008 presidential candidates' health reform proposals: choices for America. Washington, DC: The Commonwealth Fund; 2008.
4. Network for Regional Healthcare Improvement. From volume to value: transforming healthcare payment and delivery systems to improve quality and reduce costs. Pittsburgh (PA): Network for Regional Healthcare Improvement, Pittsburgh Regional Health Initiative, and Robert Wood Johnson Foundation; 2008.
5. Miller HD. From volume to value: better ways to pay for health care. Health Aff (Millwood) 2009;28(5):1418–28.
6. Robinow A. The potential of global payment: insights from the field. Washington, DC: The Commonwealth Fund; 2010.
7. Miller H. Transitioning to accountable care: incremental payment reforms to support higher quality, more affordable health care. Pittsburgh (PA): Center for Healthcare Quality and Payment Reform; 2011.
8. Hayward RA. Performance measurement in search of a path. N Engl J Med 2007; 356(9):951–95.
9. Vonnegut M. Is quality improvement improving quality? A view from the doctor's office. N Engl J Med 2007;357(26):2652–3.
10. Conway PH, Clancy C. Transformation of health care at the front line. JAMA 2009; 301(7):763–5.
11. 42 CFR Part 425 Medicare Program; Medicare Shared Savings Program: Accountable Care Organizations and Medicare Program: Waiver Designs in Connection with the Medicare Shared Savings Program and the Innovation Center; proposed rule and notice. Federal Register 2011;76 FR:19528–64.
12. Komisar HL, Feder J, Ginsburg PB. "Bundling" payment for episodes of hospital care: issues and recommendations for the New Pilot Program in Medicare. Washington, DC: Center for American Progress; 2011.
13. Centers for Medicare and Medicaid Services. Roadmap for Implementing Value Driven Healthcare into the Traditional Medicare Fee-For-Service Program. Washington, DC: Centers for Medicare and Medicaid Services; 2010.

14. 42 CFR Parts 422 and 480. Medicare Programs; Hospital Inpatient Value-Based Purchasing Program; proposed rule. Federal Register 2011;76 FR:2454–91.
15. 42 CFR Parts 410, 414, 415, and 49. Medicare Program; Payment Policies Under the Physician Fee Schedule and Other Revisions to Part B for CY 2012; proposed rule. Federal Register 2011;76 FR:42772–947.
16. Report to congress: Medicare ambulatory surgical center value-based purchasing implementation plan. Washington, DC: Department of Health and Human Services; 2011.
17. 42 CFR Parts 410, 411, 416, 419, 489, and 495. Medicare and Medicaid Programs: Hospital Outpatient Prospective Payment; Ambulatory Surgical Center Payment; Hospital Value-Based Purchasing Program; Physician Self-Referral; and Provider Agreement Regulations on Patient Notification Requirements; proposed rule. Federal Register 2011;76 FR:42170–393.
18. The Medicare Payment Advisory Committee. Physician services payment system. Washington, DC: Medicare Payment Advisory Committee; 2010.
19. 42 CFR Parts 405, 409, 410, 411, 413, 414, 415, and 424. Medicare Program; Payment Policies Under the Physician Fee Schedule and Other Revisions to Part B for CY 2011; proposed rule. Federal Register 2010;75 FR:40040–709.
20. 42 CFR Parts 405, 409, 410, 411, 413, 414, 415, and 424. Medicare Program; Payment Policies Under the Physician Fee Schedule and Other Revisions to Part B for CY 2011; final rule. Washington, DC: Federal Register 2010;75 FR:73169–860.
21. Hackbarth GM. Centers for Medicare and Medicaid Services. Letter to Donald Berwick M.D., Washington, DC: Administrator. Medicare Payment Advisory Commission; 2010.
22. 42 CFR Part 414 Medicare program; five-year review of work relative value units under the physician fee schedule; proposed rule. Federal Register 2011;76 FR: 32410–813.

The Impact of Health Care Reform on Innovation and New Technology

Robert A. Ganz, MD[a,b],*

KEYWORDS

• Innovation • Medical technology
• Food and drug administration • Venture capital

"An amazing invention but who would ever want to use one?"
—*President Rutherford B. Hayes after trying Alexander Graham Bell's telephone, patented on March 7, 1876*

"America is a country of inventors..."
—Alexander Graham Bell, 1877

Few fields have benefited more from sustained technological success than gastroenterology (GI); our patients and practices have been utterly transformed in recent years with a legion of innovation including proton-pump inhibitor therapy, the discovery of *Helicobacter pylori*, the discovery of and effective treatment for viral hepatitis, colon cancer genetics, burgeoning therapies for inflammatory bowel disease, the advent of screening colonoscopy, high-resolution manometry, and remarkable advances in endoscopic therapies including endoscopic ultrasonography, endomicroscopy with fluorescence imaging, and safe and effective ablation of Barrett esophagus, to name just a few advances. Over the past generation the United States, long the world leader in new technology and innovation, has consistently produced an impressive stream of biomedical discoveries and innovations that have saved lives, improved the quality of care for hundreds of millions of patients and, just as importantly, have helped build an enormous pharmaceutical and medical device industry that is the envy of the world in creating prosperity and hundreds of thousands of high-paying jobs. The United States currently dominates the approximately $400 billion international device industry. Of the 46 medical technology companies with more than

Disclosures: BARRX Medical, Inc—Equity holder; Torax Medical, Inc—Equity holder.
[a] Minnesota Gastroenterology, PA, Old Shakopee Road, Bloomington, MN, USA
[b] University of Minnesota, Minneapolis, MN, USA
* Minnesota Gastroenterology, PA, Old Shakopee Road, Bloomington, MN.
E-mail address: rganz@mngastro.com

Gastrointest Endoscopy Clin N Am 22 (2012) 109–120
doi:10.1016/j.giec.2011.08.006
1052-5157/12/$ – see front matter © 2012 Elsevier Inc. All rights reserved.

$1 billion in annual earnings, 32 are headquartered in the United States, accounting for roughly 40% of the global medical device market.[1]

In just the past few years, however, the general United States environment supporting this industry has greatly deteriorated, with investment in GI particularly at risk, while at the same time competing countries are moving forward in developing their own medical drug and device industries threatening our global leadership in scientific innovation (**Fig. 1**).[1] In fact, the next budding Alexander Graham Bell equivalent medical entrepreneur, who dreams of inventing the next great technology in GI, will be entering into the toughest innovation climate in recent memory. Multiple overall factors have evolved that together make this a particularly challenging time for developing new medical technologies, including the advent of health care reform with all of its uncertainties, increasingly stringent Food and Drug Administration (FDA) regulations, a tougher insurance reimbursement climate, less predictable venture funding, and the impact of the recent downturn in the economy. There are also factors unique to the field of GI that are creating specific barriers to device development in our specialty, including the practice dominance of screening colonoscopy, anticipated lower payments for endoscopic procedures, relative risk aversion, and the lack of financial incentive to pursue complex endoscopic technologies.

Why should gastroenterologists care about maintaining the United States lead in innovation, or if other countries move ahead of us in this race? For one thing, innovation and the creation of new medical value leads to better health outcomes at lower cost, and allows our patients early access to these improvements.[1] Sustaining our previous pace of medical innovation and advances in medicine can help slow and even stop the rapidly rising cost of care, particularly in societies that are rapidly aging such as the United States. The return on previous medical innovation in GI has been remarkable. To name just a few advances, the advent of screening colonoscopy has helped decrease colon cancer incidence and death rates (decreased by 13% in the last decade), better hepatitis B and C therapies have increased remission rates, and newer Barrett's ablation modalities have almost eliminated the need for esophagectomy in those with dysplasia, with vastly less morbidity and mortality.[2,3] If other countries take the lead in drug and device development, our patients, practitioners, and researchers will lose early access to these benefits, and we will fall behind in knowledge and expertise. Medical innovation drives increased productivity as well; recent gains in health and longevity are worth about $3 trillion on an annual basis in the United States.[1]

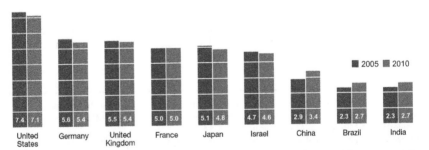

Fig. 1. Innovation scores, ranked by country (scale of 1–9, with 9 as best). Pricewaterhousecoopers (PwC) analysis from the PwC Innovation Scorecard, January 2011. (*Data from* Medical Technology Innovation Scorecard. The race for global leadership. Pricewaterhousecoopers LLC, Delaware (OH). Available at: www.pwc.com/InnovationScorecard.)

Moreover, a recent study by the Lewin Group[4] demonstrates the critical role the medical technology industry plays in the economy of the United States:

- The industry directly employed 422,778 workers
- The industry paid $24.6 billion in salaries and other earnings
- The industry shipped nearly $140 billion dollars worth of products
- Every med-tech job indirectly generated an additional 1.5 jobs and each medical technology (med-tech) dollar generated an additional $0.90 in earnings.

Thus the preservation of our dominant role in med-tech is critically important in maintaining the health and productivity of our fellow citizens, lowering our health care costs, and helping to maintain our economy. If we want to see continued progress in medicine in general and GI specifically, this is a race worth winning; however, given recent developments the long-term United States dominance of scientific innovation is no longer assured.

HEALTH CARE REFORM LEGISLATION AND INNOVATION

The Patient Protection and Affordable Care Act (PPACA) signed into law on March 23, 2010, will have an unprecedented impact on the practice of GI, and on the development of new technology in our field. The bill is enormous in scope, more than 2000 pages long, and regulations to administer the bill could run to more than 150,000 pages. The potential benefits and drawbacks of this reform legislation have been debated endlessly, and the final manifestations of the various statutes remain to be seen. The bill greatly expands access to health care, opens up Medicaid eligibility to all individuals and families with incomes up to 133% of poverty level, and also mandates health insurance exchanges intended to offer a state-by-state marketplace, where individuals and small businesses can compare policies and premiums and purchase insurance with a government subsidy, if eligibility applies. The bill eliminates all financial barriers to preexisting medical conditions and for certain preventive tests including screening colonoscopy. On its face this expansion of health insurance coverage, and elimination of barriers to screening colonoscopy, should be a boon for GI practices and also for GI pharmaceutical and device companies, because many patients previously uncovered will now have more affordable access to health care. Unfortunately however, the massive scope of the bill, the long period of time between passage and actual implementation, and the interpretation of the myriad statutes has created great uncertainties, leading to caution on the part of innovation companies. There are also statutes in the bill that may create specific barriers to innovation, and may cause less investment or a delay in the adoption of new med-tech.[5]

The health care reform legislation greatly centralizes the role of the federal and state governments, and Medicaid and Medicare payment mechanisms may dominate, particularly through the state-based exchanges. Many states are already financially strapped and as more patients enter into the Medicaid rolls, payment rates to drug and device manufacturers, physicians, and hospitals might decrease, and specific services will likely be cut. This situation has already occurred in several parts of the country, and other states are requesting Medicaid waivers and block grants that will allow them to cut or eliminate certain payments or procedures with greater facility.[6] This scenario may make it difficult for device and drug developers to recoup their costs or be profitable with new technologies. Much depends on whether the exchanges function as a robust marketplace with multiple private competing insurers, or if the government dominates with just a few federal or state-determined payers, with federal or state-mandated benefits. It is also unclear at this time whether allowed exchange benefits will be determined by third-party payers, by the federal government under Medicare, or by the individual states.

In addition, the PPACA calls for reduced annual payment updates for most Medicare and Medicaid services, substantial cuts to managed care plans, and the creation of accountable care organizations that are rewarded for holding the line on services and costs. None of this is particularly auspicious for the development and payment of new technologies. Companies may be very hesitant to develop innovations if the payment rates are too low, or if there is no mechanism to rapidly introduce the technology into a state-based or federal-based exchange plan.

Other PPACA mandates are perhaps even more concerning for the development of new technology. The bill calls for "value-based payments" for physicians, with value-payment modifiers to differentiate payments based on quality of care compared with cost, and also calls for public reporting of physician performance via a "physician compare" Web site. The Web site will include data on all patients seen, not just Medicare/Medicaid, and will also compare data between peers. In the same vein, the bill mandates the development of quality measures for each specialty. The department of Health and Human Services (HHS) in conjunction with the Agency for Healthcare Research and Quality (AHRQ), and the Centers for Medicare and Medicaid Services (CMS), is directed to develop outcomes measures for hospitals and physicians. The measures will include the 5 most prevalent and resource-intensive medical conditions per specialty. These requirements might make it difficult for physicians to rapidly introduce new technologies into practice for fear of appearing "too expensive," or using new technology and incurring initially higher complication rates.[5]

The health care reform legislation also establishes the Center for Medicare and Medicaid Innovation to "test, evaluate, and expand different payment structures and care delivery models" for providers and hospitals. Under law, the Secretary of HHS is allowed at his or her discretion to institute any payment model, including partial or full capitation, at any time and for any condition. In addition the Secretary of HHS is instructed to develop a pilot program on payment bundling for any particular disease (defined as 3 days prior to a hospital admission to 30 days post discharge), and "episode groupers," which combine clinically related items and services into an "episode of care." It is unclear whether these potential payment changes will reduce the cost of care; however, they will almost certainly introduce a chill into the introduction of new technology in GI and other specialties, because capitation and service bundling will not initially incorporate the cost of newer innovations.

The PPACA also calls for comparative effectiveness research via a Patient-Centered Outcomes Research Institute, which is instructed to look at clinical outcomes, practice variation, expenditures, and patient needs for various drugs, devices, or services. This process could also impair the introduction of newer technologies, if comparative effectiveness studies need to be completed before payments can be arranged or if this type of research increases the costs for developing new modalities.

The legislation establishes an Independent Payment Advisory Board (IPAB), a 15-member panel appointed by the President, which is intended to reduce the per capita rate of growth in Medicare spending. In the event that Medicare exceeds the expected rate of growth (which has happened almost every year since the creation of Medicare), the Board is required to make recommendations to reduce spending. By law, the IPAB is prohibited in making changes that would "ration care, raise revenues, increase premiums or modify existing benefits." Thus there is concern in some circles that the IPAB could act by reducing physician and facility fees for certain procedures, or inhibit or delay the introduction of new services and procedures in an effort to hold down costs. This situation would create significant uncertainty on the part of drug and device innovators. Not knowing if a new drug or device would be allowed, or what the payment might be for same, a company might decide to forgo development or the introduction of a new innovation. Any IPAB decision can be overridden by a two-thirds vote in Congress, but given the current political tensions between the Democrats and Republicans, this would be very difficult to achieve on any specific issue.[5]

The "Sunshine Act" is a provision of the health care legislation that requires any manufacturer of a Medicare-covered drug, device, or medical supply to report annually on any payments to physicians. The Act's provisions are draconian and apply to any payment with a value of $10 or more, or an aggregate amount greater than $100 per year. This provision will make it much more difficult for drug and device companies to market new innovations, and might also act as a drag on new development if physicians are unable to accept funding from device companies for device research or are unable to obtain money for research studies.[5]

DEVICE TAX

"If you want less of something, tax it"
                    —Milton Friedman

One of the more controversial aspects of the health care act is the excise tax on medical device companies. To pay for new health benefits for millions of those currently uninsured, the bill calls for new taxes, including a provision imposing a 2.3% tax on sales of medical devices by manufacturers, producers, and importers. The tax will begin in 2013, applies to gross revenues not net sales, and applies to those revenues generated in the United States. Taxable devices include any medical device defined in Section 201(h) of the FDA Act, and intended for use by humans, with limited exclusions for devices purchased by the general public at retail for individual use, such as eyeglasses. There is no general exclusion for Class I medical devices (bandages, gloves, tongue depressors, and so forth). The excise tax is expected to generate $20 billion from the device industry through 2019. As recently noted by the CEO of Boston Scientific, the tax will adversely affect hundreds of device companies and will specifically cost his company approximately $100 million annually. The effect of the tax will be to limit investment in innovation, as it is widely expected that this is revenue that will be taken out of research and development, thus hindering the implementation of the next generation of medical devices. GI societies can also expect less money for education and research grants as the tax bites the bottom line of endoscope and accessory manufacturers. The timing of the tax is unfortunate, as research and development as a percentage of gross domestic product (GDP) is already declining in the United States.[6] Pharmaceutical companies are also hit with a separate excise tax on drug sales, which gradually increases until the year 2019.[5,7,8]

FDA

The United States success in medical device development over recent decades has been in large measure due to a supportive regulatory and legal environment. The US FDA has been critically important in guaranteeing confidence in the safety and efficacy of our med-tech products. Unfortunately for the technology industry, however, the FDA approval process has recently come under fire for "inadequate review resources" and "poor consistency and transparency in decision-making."[9,10] In a recent survey 40% of med-tech companies experienced frequent problems in gaining product approvals, due to limited FDA resources. It now takes twice as long for the FDA to approve the same technology as it does in Europe for the 510(k) process, and complex medical devices facing the premarket approval (PMA) process will obtain approval on average 4 years earlier in Europe.[1,9,10] In another survey by Northwestern University,[11] two-thirds of small medical device manufacturers obtained approval in Europe first, and cited the FDA approval process as the reason for delaying their entry into the United States. In this survey, both large and small companies noted that unclear guidelines, inconsistent implementation, and lead reviewer turnover contributed to the increasing unpredictability of the FDA process. The majority of the respondents also stated that the European process was much more predictable than the FDA.[11]

There is concern in the device industry that the 510(k) pathway for predicate devices, typically a far quicker and more expeditious route to clearance than the more stringent PMA process, is about to become tougher. A pending report from the Institute of Medicine, regarding the 510(k) pathway, may call for FDA-approved clinical trials and more intensive review prior to approval. If adopted, these new standards could make lower-risk, predicate device approvals even more expensive and time consuming than the current already deliberate process.[12]

Although widely credited with ensuring patient safety, the increasing uncertainty of the FDA approval process is causing disruption in the United States technology industry for several reasons. There is a "brain drain" as new devices and resources migrate to Europe, and companies experience much more difficulty in attracting investors at a reasonable price. Any uncertainty in the FDA process leads to the need for additional studies and time to complete them, which in turn leads to a longer, more expensive, and uncertain cost proposition. All of these factors will lead to less innovation, less competitiveness for United States companies, and loss of opportunity to overseas markets. A rising number of companies, especially those backed by venture-capital financing, are choosing to launch new medical technologies abroad rather than wait for the FDA approval in the United States first.[9,11]

It is not widely appreciated among gastroenterologists how the much tougher FDA regulatory policies profoundly affect the general United States med-tech industry, and how these policies can limit our access to new technology and also to investment in the GI field. Several promising GI devices are only available in Europe as they await FDA approval, such as the Pillcam for colon cancer screening, the Torax Magnetic Sphincter LINX antireflux device, and several antiobesity devices including the Intra-Pace gastric pacemaker, the GI Dynamics Endobarrier small intestinal sleeve device, and several newer gastric balloons. The field of obesity devices has been particularly problematic with regard to FDA policies, because the agency has been dilatory in releasing their standards and there is no current clear path to FDA approval. Some obesity companies such as Satiety (endoscopic vertical banded gastroplasty), which raised $80 million in venture financing, have recently failed because they could not overcome difficult FDA hurdles.[13] Other obesity companies have not been able to reach agreement with the FDA on the clinical trials needed to win approval, because the FDA has not yet determined the absolute weight loss necessary, nor specified the difference needed in comparison with a control group. Some company executives have been told they need a difference in weight loss between a device and control group of 25%, which is more than that achieved by the Lap-Band when it was approved! It must be noted that the Lap-Band, a surgical procedure with a relatively high adverse event profile, was also approved without a control group or randomized trial design, which is now deemed necessary. These FDA-related uncertainties and more difficult standards will make the investment community more hesitant to invest in the GI space in the United States, decreasing the device opportunities for ourselves and our patients.[13]

REIMBURSEMENT FOR NEW TECHNOLOGY

No country in the world spends as much on a per capita basis for health care as does the United States, roughly $8000 per person per year.[1] We spend about 19% of our GDP on medical care, nearly 50% more than most countries in the world (**Fig. 2**). Although expensive, and yielding uncertain health benefits beyond what most countries expend, this enormous health care market provides ready access for the adoption of new technology and entices new companies to innovate. Moreover, Americans typically pay little out of pocket for health care; the patient share of total health expenditures declined from 47% in 1960 to 12% today.[14] The historical structure of American health care, with almost all costs paid by a third-party insurer or the government, have rendered us largely unaware of the cost of treatment with little resistance to demand for the latest and greatest therapy, service, or drug. Traditionally then, the doctor has been the arbiter of new value in technology, with insurers and the government passively absorbing the costs, the patients actively demanding services without limit, and little resistance to the introduction and adoption of new innovations.

However, with the advent of ever-rising health care costs, economic doldrums from the "great recession," and the health care reform legislation, this old dynamic is disappearing and the patient share of costs is rapidly rising. More employers are forcing increasingly higher deductibles, copayments, and limitations of coverage onto employees. A recent Kaiser Family Foundation survey found that 46% of small employers required workers to pay annual deductibles of at least $1000.[15] As patients shell out more out of pocket they are increasingly resistant to pay for expensive new drugs and procedures.

At the same time, health care reform legislation and the insurance industry as a whole are putting the spotlight on "value" as opposed to volume of services. Insurers and the government are now demanding higher value at lower cost, and also demanding that new procedures be compared with existing technology to

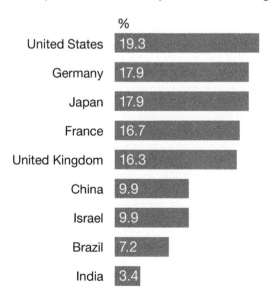

Fig. 2. Expenditure on health care by country. World Health Organization data from 2006, PwC analysis. (*Data from* Medical Technology Innovation Scorecard. The race for global leadership. PricewaterhouseCoopers LLC, Delaware (OH). Available at: www.pwc.com/ InnovationScorecard.)

demonstrate real improvement as opposed to incremental benefit. Third-party payers are disinclined to pay for "me-too" products that are incrementally better but also more expensive. In most cases, they are also demanding rigorous trials with measurable end points for any new innovations. This situation is creating new strain on innovation companies and their financiers as the path to payment approval now often requires multiple, expensive, prospective, randomized, controlled studies with long-term follow-up.

Under the new health care reform legislation, the pressure on insurance companies to hold down costs, for example, hold down expenditures for new technology, will be enormous. Under the new bill, insurers are prohibited from imposing lifetime dollar limits on essential benefits (ie, hospital stays and so forth), dependent children are allowed to remain on their parents' insurance plan until age 26 years, insurers are prohibited from excluding preexisting medical conditions, are prohibited from charging copayments or deductibles for certain preventive care and medical screenings, cannot enforce annual spending caps, and are prohibited from dropping policyholders when they get sick. All of these provisions and new coverage requirements will prove to be extremely expensive for third-party payers, and in order to cover these new requirements they will be much more discerning and resistant to paying for any new services.[5]

In addition, the federal health law is aimed at making sure that third-party payers are not able to set their premiums too much above their costs. federal and state regulators are increasingly scrutinizing the rate requests of all insurers as a direct result of the health reform legislation, and are also being very discerning regarding insurance company profits. The law allows for state-by-state review of insurance rates, a process that will closely monitor insurance company profits. For example, BCBS of California, a large nonprofit health insurer, has recently come under criticism for its double-digit rate increases. Under pressure from federal and state regulators as well as consumer groups, the company pledged to limit its profit to no more than 2% of its revenue, and also planned to return $180 million of profit the company made above its 2010 target. In previous years that extra profit would likely be plowed back into paying for new technology, but now under pressure, this insurer and others will return extra money to its clients. Although this may benefit clients in the short run, in the long run the adoption new technology may suffer as a result.[16]

An additional barrier to insurance reimbursement for innovation is the advent of technology assessment boards such as the California Technology Assessment Forum, an extension of the insurance industry, which influences the various BCBS companies, and whose decisions affect roughly 90 million covered insurance lives in the United States. Other boards such as ECRI and Hayes, Inc offer independent, albeit still quite stringent, assessments of new innovation. In the past, GI societies and journals would largely direct the application and uses of new GI innovations, but that power is rapidly shifting to outside assessment such as already noted. These various assessment boards provide approvals or disapprovals of new technology, comparative effectiveness reviews, and clinical guideline development, and determine whether or not technology should be paid for and under what circumstances the devices can be used. This change represents a serious shift in clinical power, not yet fully appreciated by the GI community or the GI societies, which are at risk to be rendered increasingly irrelevant in the clinical practice arena. If the GI societies and their members want to maintain relevance in this arena, they will need to increasingly assert themselves in the support of new GI technology.

Many new small GI technology companies have already discovered how difficult the new reimbursement landscape has become. Due to higher insurance barriers or unrealistic assessment board reviews, FDA-approved GI devices such as SmartPill, the Pillcam Eso, and the Halo Barrett's ablation technology either cannot garner consistent insurance coverage or are limited to treatment of certain conditions. Lack of, or incomplete, insurance coverage can hinder these techniques before they reach their full clinical potential, and may also limit the ability to conduct evaluation trials or generate improved next-generation products. These coverage issues will also be a disincentive for further investment in our specialty.

VENTURE-CAPITAL FINANCING

None of the myriad aforementioned issues has been lost on the investment community, which has turned increasingly sour on medical technology investments. United States venture-capital investment in medical technology has dropped substantially over the past several years (**Fig. 3**).[1] There has been a significant shakeout going on in the venture industry over the past 3 to 4 years; the United States has gone from more than 1000 venture firms in 2007 to fewer than 400 today, and the United States now ranks fourth in the world in terms of medical entrepreneurial activity behind the emerging nations China, Brazil, and India.[1,17] The economic turmoil of recent years and the accompanying slump in the stock market have been major factors hurting the industry, with negative 10-year returns on venture-capital investments. Moreover, the current environment of increasingly stringent and uncertain FDA requirements, clinical trial risks, market adoption and reimbursement questions, and constrained exit options decreases predictability in investment success for new ventures.

In addition, the new health care reform act introduces new uncertainty about the federal and individual state government process for reviewing new products. The initial public offering (IPO) market has been hurt by these issues and is no longer particularly receptive to medical device companies. Venture capitalists are sensitive to the time required to get a return on their investment and are increasingly reluctant

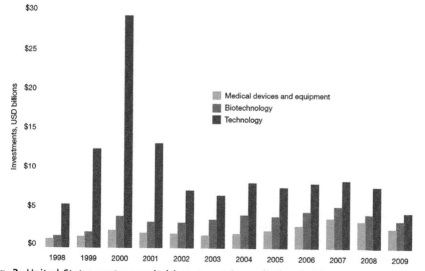

Fig. 3. United States venture-capital investment in medical technology. National Venture Capital Association report 2010; PwC analysis. (*Data from* Medical Technology Innovation Scorecard. The race for global leadership. PricewaterhouseCoopers LLC, Delaware (OH). Available at: www.pwc.com/InnovationScorecard.)

to place money in medical startups that that take much longer to exit in comparison with previous eras. Medical technology deals now take an average of 10 years to have an exit or liquidity event, via either IPO or acquisition by a larger company, up from 4 to 5 years in the earlier part of the decade.[18] Going forward, if this trend line in fewer venture-capital companies and decreased investment continues, we can anticipate less, and more cautious, funding of GI startups with less development in the field. We can also anticipate much of the early, new GI technology moving overseas for initial testing and adoption.

GI-SPECIFIC ISSUES

There are several issues unique to current GI practice that make our specialty less attractive to investors in new technology. On a demographic basis, we are a rapidly aging specialty, with the average age of practicing gastroenterologists now greater than 50. This aging is a significant problem because older physicians tend to be less aggressive, less likely to learn new skills and adopt new technology, and less likely to perform endoscopic research and publish. In addition, we are likely training too few GI fellows for the clinical needs of the country, especially if, as expected, about one-third of current practitioners retire within the next 10 years.[19,20]

At the same time, our aging and manpower issues have been greatly exacerbated by the upsurge in procedural volumes with the advent of screening colonoscopy. As our practices and practice economics become increasingly dominated by screening colonoscopy, we have less time for cognitive services, and less time or financial inclination to research or incorporate new innovations. As a result, the adoption and acceptance of new technology will quite likely be slower than in the past, with fewer willing "early adopters." Moreover, to be economically competitive with existing practice any new endoscopic innovations will be forced to fit into the current practice paradigm, that is, take less than half an hour to perform, and be simple, safe, and easy to learn. These implications are unattractive for GI device manufacturers, who will be increasingly prone to introduce complex new techniques outside the United States.[19,20]

Given the expectations of the health care reform legislation, it is widely anticipated that payment for GI services and procedures will be even more centralized than today, and quite likely that current endoscopic payment will either remain the same or decline slightly. We are also very likely to see more capitated payment models, that is, bundling and payment for episodes of care. This trend is not auspicious for device development because payment for increasingly more complex endoscopic procedures will remain relatively low, and users of time-intensive complex techniques will be penalized by bundling. Thus the expected payment system will reward the performance of relatively simple cases or reward not performing cases at all. All of this will lead to less profit for GI device manufacturers, fewer interested corporate parties, and potentially less overall future development and investment in the field.[19,20]

THE FUTURE

This article has reviewed many of the threats to the development of new innovation and new technology, in medicine in general and to GI specifically. Are these issues preordained or can gastroenterologists influence our future access to new technology and preserve our practices and future? Much remains unknown; however, it is clear that we cannot do things as we have in the past and expect a sanguine outcome. Gastroenterologists and the GI societies need to recognize that our power to shape our clinical practices is rapidly being lost to insurance companies intent on holding the bottom line, non-GI technology assessment boards with no clinical experience or intimate knowledge of GI practice, an increasingly more difficult FDA regulatory landscape, and governmental agencies that will increasingly call the tune as to what constitutes "value" and dictate what we can and cannot do. We will also be at the mercy of an increasingly competitive venture-capital market that might well choose to invest in other specialties or invest in other countries.

We must acknowledge the various issues at hand and urgently start to consider effective options for securing our technological future. This approach might entail any number of strategies beyond the scope of the present article, but we must recognize that if we want new technology in GI it will no longer come easily: we will have to fight for it.

REFERENCES

1. Medical Technology Innovation Scorecard. The race for global leadership. Delaware (OH). PricewaterhouseCoopers LLC. Available at: www.pwc.com/Innovation Scorecard. Accessed July 15, 2011.
2. Richardson LC, Tai E. Centers for disease control. Morb Mortal Wkly Rep 2011; 60:1–6.
3. Shaheen NJ, Sharma P, Overholt BF, et al. Radiofrequency ablation in Barrett's esophagus with dysplasia. N Engl J Med 2009;360:2277–88.
4. The Lewin Group. State economic impact of the medical technology industry. Available at: www.socalbio.org/studies/MTI_Lewin_2010. Accessed July 15, 2011.
5. Available at: http://en.wikipedia.org/wiki/Patient_Protection_and_Affordable_Care_Act. Accessed July 15, 2011.
6. Deep Medicaid cuts suddenly on table in North Carolina. Available at: http://www.newsobserver.com/2011. Accessed July 15, 2011.
7. Elliott R. A tax that arrived with the health care law impedes industry. Minneapolis (MN): Star Tribune; 2011. Section A, p. 9.
8. Pipes S. Cut health care costs: bet on medical research. New York City: Forbes, Inc; 2011. p. 16.
9. California Healthcare Institute. Competitiveness and regulation: the FDA and the future of America's biomedical industry. 2011. Available at: www.chi.org/uploadedFiles/Industry_at_glance/Competitiveness_and_Regulation. Accessed July 15, 2011.
10. Lee J. FDA under fire. Chicago (IL): Modern Healthcare Inc; 2011. p. 16.
11. Northwestern survey finds FDA predictability a top concern among medtech firms. Available at: www.inhealth.org/wtn/Page.asp?PageID=WTN004937. Accessed July 15, 2011.
12. Meier B. Study of medical device rules is attacked. New York City: New York Times Inc; 2011.
13. Pollack A. Hoping to avoid the knife. New York City: New York Times Inc; 2011.
14. CMS, National health expenditures data, historical. Available at: www.cms.gov/NationalHealthExpendData/02_NationalHealthAccountsHistorical.asp. Accessed July 15, 2011.
15. Kaiser Family Foundation News Release. Family health premiums rise 3 percent, but worker's share jumps 14 percent as firms shift cost burden, September 2nd, 2010. Available at: www.kff.org/insurance/090210nr.cfm. Accessed July 15, 2011.
16. Abelson R. California insurer says it will cap earnings. New York City: New York Times Inc; 2011.
17. Gobry PE. Over half of VC firms have shut down. Business insider. Available at: www.businessinsider.com/death-of-venture-capital-2011-2. Accessed July 15, 2011.

18. Ferrari R. Medtech venture capital heads into unfamiliar terrain. Start-up Philadelphia (PA): WB Saunders; 2008. p. 30–6.
19. Ganz R. The development and implementation of new endoscopic technology—what are the challenges? Gastrointest Endosc 2004;60:592–8.
20. Ganz R. Gastroenterology practice in 2006; challenges and opportunities. Gastrointest Endosc Clin N Am 2006;16:611–21.

The Gastroenterologist and Industry: Changing Winds

Mark H. DeLegge, MD

KEYWORDS

• Industry • Conflict of interest • Pharmaceutical industry
• Medical device industry • Physician education

The professional practice of medicine is constantly changing. One only needs to review alterations in medical school education, residency work hours, physician recredentialing, and the development of physician scorecards to realize the degree of change.[1] Because every dollar of health care spending is being scrutinized, many past relationships in health care are being evaluated for value and cost-effectiveness. An example of this is the relationships between professional physician organizations, physicians, and industry.

WHAT IS THE PROBLEM?

In 2004, members of a research team published the first national survey of physician-industry relationships (PIRs), in which 94% of respondents reported at least 1 type of industry relationship.[2] However, these relationships are varied. The 2004 study showed that receiving prescription samples or food in the workplace was reported most frequently, and reimbursement for the costs of medical meetings or continuing education, as well as speaking and consulting fees, were common.

In 2010, a similar national survey was repeated.[3] A stratified random sample of 2938 primary care physicians (internal medicine, family practice, and pediatrics) and specialists (cardiology, general surgery, psychiatry, and anesthesiology) were approached. A total of 1891 physicians completed the survey, yielding an overall response rate of 64.4%. The main outcome measurement was prevalence of PIRs and comparison with PIRs reported in 2004. The results of the 2010 study showed that, overall, 83.8% of all respondents reported some type of relationship with industry during the previous year, a 10% decline from 94% in 2004. Of those with PIRs:

63.8% received drug samples, down from 78% in 2004
70.8% received food and beverages, down from 83% in 2004

Financial disclosures: Cook Medical; Baxter Healthcare; Coram Healthcare; Apria Healthcare; DeLegge Medical.
Digestive Disease Center, Medical University of South Carolina, DeLegge Medical, 25 Courtenay Street, Suite 7100A, Charleston, SC 29425, USA
E-mail address: deleggem@musc.edu

Gastrointest Endoscopy Clin N Am 22 (2012) 121–134
doi:10.1016/j.giec.2011.08.002
1052-5157/12/$ – see front matter © 2012 Elsevier Inc. All rights reserved.

18.3% received reimbursements, including continuing medical education (CME), down from 35% in 2004

14.1% said they had been given payments for serving on advisory boards and enrolling patients in clinical trials, compared with 28% in 2004.

The 2010 study also found that the number of meetings respondents reported having with pharmaceutical company representatives decreased from an average of 3 a month to 2 a month. The investigators noted that this change could reflect greater pressures on a physician's time as well as institutional policy changes.

Cardiologists were most likely to report industry relationships, whereas psychiatrists (a specialty not included in the earlier survey) were the least likely. Physicians in solo, 2-person, or group practices were more likely to receive drug samples, meeting reimbursements, or gifts than those in hospitals and medical schools, but academically based physicians were most likely to receive payments for speaking, consulting, or serving on advisory boards.

Although the landscape of PIRs has changed significantly since 2004, many physicians still value their work and collaboration with industry. The author of these 2 studies noted that, although "physician-industry relationships have decreased significantly since 2004, they are still found among more than three-quarters of those responding to our survey." He asserted that, based on "the persistence of industry's substantial financial interaction with U.S. physicians, there is a need for a nationwide system to publicly report these relationships."[3]

ProPublica and Consumer Reports performed a survey investigating patients' perspectives regarding physicians who accept Pharmaceutical Research and Manufacturers Association (PhRMA) payments.[4] The survey indicates that patients are largely unaware of the nature of physician/PhRMA contacts, and 74% of survey respondents disapproved of physicians taking payments for promoting medications to other physicians. Furthermore, 95% of respondents noted that their physicians had not disclosed any PhRMA payments, and 70% thought that physicians should disclose that information. The survey shows that most (51%) respondents thought that payments as low as $500 could influence a physician's judgment.

WHAT STANCE HAVE ACADEMIC MEDICAL CENTERS TAKEN?

The current trend of academic medical centers (AMCs) and professional organizations to adopt policies that restrict and/or police permissible interactions and activities between industry and physicians originated from a set of recommendations proposed by Brennan and colleagues[5] in 2006. The proposed policies placed restrictions on faculty, residents, students, and staff that prohibit the receiving of gifts, samples, and many other activities.

One of the main reasons AMCs began to adopt these policies was as an attempt to avoid financial conflicts of interest that could compromise core values of altruism and fiduciary relationships. They propose that profit motives and financial gains unavoidably introduce bias in medical decision making and violate public trust, which suggests that profit is not a value that should be held by clinicians. However, many clinicians admit that the reality of their employment and pay is determined by the profitability of an AMC or a private entity.[6]

WHAT ABOUT CLINICIAN EDUCATION WITH INDUSTRY?

In today's rapidly changing medical environment, health care practitioners in every area, including gastroenterology, depend on new clinical information and data to learn about breakthroughs in science and medical technology.[7] Although some health care practitioners can learn about such breakthroughs from colleagues or attendance at major medical meetings, and others can read about them in journals, most practitioners are simply time limited or resource limited in their ability to find the pertinent information to help them improve their skills and knowledge.

Local CME is an option for health care practitioners to learn about new information and updates to guidelines and best practices in specific clinical areas.[8] These local events may be sponsored by a local university, medical society or other qualified CME organization. The local aspects of these events can avoid the cost and time associated with traveling to a meeting. In other situations, some practitioners choose purely commercial events, sponsored by a specific pharmaceutical or medical device company, to learn about a new product, treatment, use, or indication. Other health care practitioners learn about new drugs and treatments by participating in research sponsored in part or entirely by the pharmaceutical industry. The Internet has provided many on-line programs for education, some CME approved, others either sponsored by industry or individual clinicians.[9]

Throughout all of these interactions, health care practitioners depend on a certain level of interaction with industry. The clinician-industry relationship is essential for many reasons and, without it, transmission of medical information, development and improvement in medical products, and advancements in patient care could be hampered.

WHERE SHOULD THE CLINICIAN AND INDUSTRY MARKETING INTERSECT?

One of the types of physician-industry interactions that have been heavily criticized in the past several years is product marketing.[10] Many anti-industry critics believe that pharmaceutical and medical device companies use marketing techniques, marketing representatives, and other mechanisms to influence the clinical decisions and prescribing behavior of health care practitioners. Although there were abuses in the past, such as discussing the off-label use of products with physicians, the provision of lavish free meals and inappropriate gifts, kickbacks for product use, and consulting fees directly tied to a product's use, times have changed significantly since then and such behaviors today are now limited. Policies enacted by PhRMA (**Box 1**) and AdvaMed (**Box 2**) have placed strict bans on gift giving, and numerous regulations from the US Food and Drug Administration (FDA), Health and Human Services (HHS), Department of Justice (DOJ), and Office of the Inspector General (OIG) have made the risk and penalty for any illegal behaviors severe.[11] The enforcement of such rules in the past several years has increased greatly through efforts to eliminate fraud and abuse in government programs such as Medicare and Medicaid.[12]

However, the controversy in this area persists with passionate feelings aligned on both sides of the debate. An example of this is an article published by Brody and Light[13] in the American Journal of Public Health proposing a concept known as the pharmaceutical inverse benefit law.

According to the investigators, this inverse benefit law shows how pharmaceutical marketing affects the clinician decision-making process when prescribing medications. A summary of the article in the Journal of the American Medical Association summarized the law and explained that the "law was inspired by the inverse square law of physics."[14] This law suggests that there are 6 marketing strategies that create an environment in which prescribing certain drugs could undermine, rather than promote, patient safety and public health. These 6 proposed marketing strategies are:

- Reducing thresholds for diagnosing disease. For example, type II diabetes guidelines have gradually reduced the blood glucose threshold at which diabetes

---

Box 1
Key points of PhRMA guidelines

- Prohibits distribution of noneducational items (such as pens or mugs, typically adorned with a company or product logo) to health care providers and their staff.
- Gifts deemed to be educational items may not exceed $100 in value.
- Prohibits company sales representatives from providing restaurant meals to health care professionals, but allows them to provide occasional meals in health care professionals' offices in conjunction with informational presentations.
- Companies may continue to sponsor CME if the following guidelines are met:
  - Any financial support should be given to the CME provider, which, in turn, can use the money to reduce the overall CME registration fee for all participants.
  - The CME provider should follow standards for commercial support established by the Accreditation Council for Continuing Medical Education (ACCME) or another entity that may accredit the CME.
  - The company should not provide any advice or guidance to the CME provider.
  - The company may not offer direct or indirect financial support to cover the costs of travel, lodging, or other personal expenses of nonfaculty health care professionals attending CME.
  - Financial assistance for scholarships or other educational funds to permit medical students, residents, fellows, and other health care professionals in training to attend carefully selected educational conferences may be offered if the selection of individuals who will receive the funds is made by the academic or training institution.
- Companies may continue to obtain the services of professional consultants who provide advisory services if certain criteria for a bona fide consulting arrangement are met.
- Companies should require any health care professional who is a member of a committee that sets formularies or develops clinical guidelines and also serves as a speaker or commercial consultant for the company to disclose to the committee the existence and nature of his or her relationship with the company.
- Companies that choose to use non–patient-identified prescriber data to facilitate communications with health care professionals should use the data responsibly.

---

should be diagnosed and medically treated despite a lack of evidence that tight control improves major outcomes.

- Relying on surrogate end points. When physicians accept surrogate end points rather than improved clinical outcomes as goals of therapy, fewer patients need to be treated with a drug or a device to show an improved outcome, even though that outcome may not directly benefit the patient.
- Exaggerating safety claims. By overemphasizing the safety of a new drug that has been used in few patients, marketers encourage physicians to prescribe the medication to an expanded population of patients with milder symptoms, thereby exposing larger numbers of individuals to the drug and, therefore, to the potential for adverse events.
- Exaggerating efficacy claims. When an expensive new drug performs no better than established lower-cost therapies but may have an advantage for a small subset of a patient population, marketers emphasize the latter to imply that the new drug is better than an established therapy.
- Creating new diseases. For example, the invention of the disease categories of prehypertension and prediabetes potentially expands the patient population to

---

Box 2
Key points of the AdvaMed guidelines

Hospitality, meals and receptions, and spouses. Industry-sponsored hospitality is limited to modest meals and receptions for health care professionals attending sales and promotional meetings, third-party conferences, and member-sponsored product training and education. Travel or hospitality for spouses and guests overall is prohibited, although travel for health care professionals attending these meetings is allowed within certain guidelines.

Third-party conferences. Only health care providers in training can receive scholarships that are underwritten by grants from medical technology companies. The training institution or the conference sponsor, not the medical technology company, must select the scholarship recipients. Medical technology companies may not select or pay for conference speakers.

Gifts. Medical technology firms may provide modest, occasional gifts to health care professionals if they benefit the patient or serve a genuine educational function and have a fair market value of less than $100 (textbooks and anatomic models excepted).

Research and other grants. Companies may make donations for a charitable purpose, such as supporting genuine independent medical research for the advancement of medical science or education, indigent care, patient education, public education, or the sponsorship of events where proceeds are intended for charitable purposes.

Consulting services: It is appropriate to reasonably compensate health care professionals for performing bona fide consulting services, as defined by the AdvaMed code. For example, the agreements must be in writing, provide for fair market value compensation, and be entered into only if a legitimate need and purpose is identified in advance. Selection of consultants should be based solely on the consultant's qualifications and expertise to address the identified purpose.

---

be treated medically. However, this approach requires treating much larger numbers of persons to benefit a few.

- Encouraging unapproved uses. Because promoting unapproved uses of a drug is illegal, some marketers have used tactics such as manipulating the content of CME programs, hiring leading physicians to give presentations recommending off-label use.

However, critics of this article note that the investigators provide no evidence of how often this occurs and include no evidence of harm to patients from this subtle manipulation. There was no economic number placed on these subtle manipulations. Critics also note that, although there have been abuses in the past, which may correspond with some of the marketing principles listed earlier, these abuses are rare and are handled and corrected through legal and regulatory actions. In addition, critics state that the proposed efforts to nullify these marketing effects, although potentially creating a safety net to penalize the worse offenders, creates more unnecessary confusion about what kind of information physicians can receive from the industry marketing arena and could potentially harm patients when physicians refuse to look at studies or research or collaborate with industry for fear of subtle manipulation. These critics also note that Americans are generally not living longer today because of a better diet and exercise; they are living longer because there are medications and devices that prevent and treat disease. Overcorrection of the clinician-industry relationship could significantly impair important advances in medicine.

WHAT IS THE STANCE OF THE ASSOCIATION OF AMERICAN MEDICAL COLLEGES?

The Association of American Medical Colleges (AAMC) recently considered a task force report on developing guidelines to manage PIRs.[15] This report recommends, among other things, the development of policies that prohibit all gifts from industry for physicians, faculty, staff, students, and trainees of AMCs, either on-site or off-site. The report also recommends that the prohibition apply to equipment and service vendors.

According to the report, medical centers should discourage their faculty, students, and trainees from:

- Attending nonaccredited industry events that are marketed as CME
- Accepting payment for attendance at industry-sponsored meetings
- Accepting gifts from industry representatives at meetings
- Participating in ghostwriting.

Further, the task force recommends that pharmaceutical representatives not be permitted access to patient care areas, that device representative visits be limited to those who are appropriately credentialed, and that such visits be only at the request of a physician.

The ramifications of the AAMC policy are evident in the current degree of oversight of pharmaceutical and device manufacturer interaction with clinicians on a local level. An example of this is the Conflict of Interest in Clinical Care – Policy on Pharmaceutical and Medical Device Relationship from the University of Washington, St Louis, Missouri.[16] This policy noted that pharmaceutical and medical device representatives have an interest in making health care professionals aware of their products and new product developments. They noted that, although interactions with sales representatives have a legitimate purpose, it is essential that information provided by these individuals is free of bias and financial inducements that might unduly influence medical decision making. The purpose of the policy was to define ethical standards for interacting with pharmaceutical and medical device manufacturers. This policy defined these clinician-industry relationships as follows:

1. Vendor sales representatives are allowed on Washington University School of Medicine (WUSM) premises only by appointment and only in department-designated areas as approved by the Department Chair, Program Director, or their respective designees.
2. Vendor sales representatives are prohibited from having direct patient contact. Any exceptions to this policy must be approved by the Department Chair or Program Director and limited to situations in which the presence of a medical device representative is essential because of the complexity of the medical device being used.
3. Pharmaceutical/medical device manufacturers may only provide unrestricted educational grants to a central fund with the approval of the Department Chair, Program Director, or their respective designees. The fund is independent of any industry input or control.
4. Grants may be used for medical education purposes including, but not limited to, medical textbooks, honoraria, and expenses for extramural lecturers and the provision of modest food/meals.
5. Grants cannot be conditional or related in any way to any preexisting or future business relationship with the industrial sponsor.
6. The content of the educational program and related materials must be under the exclusive control of WUSM.
7. Financial support of programs can be acknowledged in text in program announcements (eg, "This program was supported in part by an educational grant from ....").

8. When industry provides support of CME-accredited educational activities, additional CME guidelines and procedures for commercial support of educational activities must be followed.
9. Educational events may be publicized if supported by an unrestricted educational grant.

These policies are not the most restrictive among academic centers. There is recognition from AMCs that industry representatives may be needed by clinicians during the use of complicated medical devices. Many AMCs rely on a pool of money to be used as deemed fit by the Department Chair or Program Director for education events and other industry-related activities. This pooled funding may seem logical but may jeopardize industry-sponsored CME programs if companies cannot justify the expense of donating monies that may serve the greater good but have no relationship to a company's future success and future ability to contribute funds for medical education. In addition, most AMCs have not taken the initiative in providing their own postgraduate physicians with the training and education in and on complicated medical devices or complicated medical therapy that results in increased hospital reputation, increased hospital profit, and improved patient care.

WHAT ARE THE ISSUES FOR PROFESSIONAL MEDICAL SOCIETIES?

Professional medical societies have been criticized in the last few years for the way they handle commercial funds for medical education.[17] They have distanced themselves from industry by using third parties as a neutral buffer to organize and operationalize continuing education programs. Some critics have suggested using pooled industry funds to decrease suspicion of the impact of industry on the science of medicine, which has led to several suggestions for how to use commercial funds to support medical education activities.

Executives from the American Gastroenterological Association Institute (AGAI) have proposed setting up a corporate education fund (CEF) to take aggregated contributions for Independent Medical Education conferences.[18] This would consist of a pooled fund of money from multiple industry partners to be used by the American Gastroenterological Association (AGA) as deemed necessary irrespective of the education programs goals. Under this proposal, an AGA education committee would decide curriculum topics and learning methods. All activities would offer CME credit and would meet all ACCME and PhRMA guidelines and requirements. Unlike an endowment, CEF monies would be spent and replenished annually. The hope was that this fund would refute the perception that any direct funding of an educational activity is tainted no matter what steps are taken. The aggregated money could also be used to fund CME programs that would otherwise not get funded because they lack commercial interest.

However, this is a difficult challenge for industry. Margins for profit in the health care industry have fallen substantially and future health care law and directions seem likely to further restrict pricing.[19] Many believe that the days of asking companies to provide associations or clinicians money for education with no concern for their therapeutic area or business interest are long gone. Some believe that pharmaceutical or device companies would be loathe to award grants for programs that do not align with their interests.

Ultimately, with various policies in place, such as the ACCME Standards for Commercial Support, PhRMA and AdvaMed codes of ethics, and other rules and regulations from HHS, OIG, and FDA, the idea of a generic pool for CME funding is probably too late, too restrictive, and unnecessary. Supporters of avoiding stricter CME oversight would note that industry and commercial medical education and medical affairs departments review detailed proposals that address specific areas of medicine. As a result, it may be that the current structure of commercial support of CME funding is more than adequate to address any potential issues that critics may identify.

The continued support of CME by industry is important. Medical professional societies have ethical, positive relationships with industry, as do others in federal and state government and the foundation community. Public funding is limited, particularly in the current economic climate, for education, quality initiatives, and research. Foundation and other such philanthropic support can only go so far. Without continued external support from industry, many societies may be unable to provide the same level of outstanding education and cutting-edge science that has advanced the quality of patient care in this country. Moreover, as funding and reimbursements are tightened, medical practices and practitioners are likely to lag further behind in obtaining the most current, evidence-based information as the pace of scientific progress accelerates.

HOW IMPORTANT ARE INDUSTRY RELATIONSHIPS TO PROFESSIONAL MEDICAL SOCIETIES?

The importance of the professional medical society-industry relationship can be noted in a joint press conference with the AGA, American College of Cardiology, the American College of Emergency Room Physicians, the American College of Radiologists, the American College of Rheumatology, and the American Society of Plastic Surgeons in April 2009.[20] All these societies stated that they are committed to the highest ethical standards. They also stated that they strive for responsible, transparent relationships in which industry support has no influence on educational content, quality measures, or scientific research. They note that these individual societies adhere to the ACCME standards and that each society has stringent internal policies in place to ensure that their educational and scientific content remains unbiased. These societies noted that their industry supporters adhere to guidelines from PhRMA and the Advanced Medical Technology Association (AdvaMed). The society group professed its commitment to 5 major principles: transparency, patient centeredness, active management of conflicts of interest, accountability, and reporting. These societies also underscored that industry interactions with health care professionals are critical and designed to enhance the practice of medicine and benefits to patients.

THE MEDICAL DEVICE INDUSTRY

The medical device industry and clinicians have had an intimate association in the past 50 years. The expansion of new medical device technology has been as a result of great ideas, generally starting with a clinician in a particular field collaborating with bioengineers of small and large corporations.[21] Although the dynamics of how medical devices are approved on the regulatory side have changed in the past 2 decades, as has the amount of investment to bring a new product to the market, the uniqueness and importance of the clinician-bioengineer relationship remains a pivotal step in the development of new medical technology.

Recently, the Society of American Gastrointestinal and Endoscopic Surgeons (SAGES) made some strong statements about the clinician-industry relationships concerning medical devices.[22] They noted that congress and others have called into question the propriety of professional medical associations (PMAs), clinicians, and industry relationships.[17,23] However, SAGES considers these relationships to be critical to the continued development of new and better surgical devices and procedures for patients. They stated that "the importance of clinicians in the development of medical devices cannot be overstated." In addition, they noted that PMAs should work with industry in defined ways to educate physicians about new procedures and devices. The involvement of physicians and PMAs with the development and deployment of new drugs, tools, and procedures has been integral to the progress realized by the medical profession in providing safer, higher-quality care to patients; this is especially true in the development of medical instruments.

SAGES further detailed several important points that must be highlighted when considering the issue of regulating the relationships between industry and individual physicians or PMAs. They are:

- The medical device industry and the pharmaceutical industry are different in their approach to the development of new products.
- The medical device development industry is essential to physician innovation and development of new technology.
- Research and development and education must be differentiated and separated from industry sales and marketing.
- Full disclosure and complete transparency of physician financial relationships with industry are critical.

Pharmaceutical products are often developed by researchers employed directly by the company or through an academic or commercial laboratory; a process often devoid of the practicing physician's direct involvement. The pharmaceutical company expends considerable in-house resources before the drug is available for potential clinical use. Only after the drug is fully developed does the practicing physician use the drug in pharmaceutical industry–directed drug trials to establish safety and efficacy. Clinical research involves compensation to the investigators, investigator's laboratories, and their institution that covers direct costs, research overheads, and possibly some surplus (or loss) in return for their participation in such trials. At this point in the development of a new drug, the company has considerable incentive to see the drug reach the market so that they can recover their significant up-front investment, which can range from $800 million to nearly $2 billion per drug.[24] In this setting, there may be an expectation that the physician's role is more focused on confirmation of the company's claims and publication of satisfactory results, and less so on the development or refinement of the drug.

In contrast, a medical device company rarely develops an instrument with in-house resources alone, but relies on individual physicians to bring forward clinical needs and concepts for devices. Physicians often actively participate with in-house engineers (who are not clinicians) to both develop and improve products.[21] Device companies do not maintain a substantial in-house staff of scientists and researchers but instead they employ engineers who can translate the ideas and needs of practicing physicians into instrument prototypes. Thus, the device company's resources are more heavily leveraged toward identifying and exploring clinical needs as defined by procedure-oriented physicians such as surgeons or endoscopists, and refining prototypes of tools to meet established clinical needs. It is this direct relationship with the physician that allows the development and advancement of medical procedures, often resulting in less-invasive procedures that directly benefit patients. Device companies and their engineers cannot independently develop instruments for medical care.

SAGES also notes that PMAs have a particularly important role to play in the process of educating and training physicians in the use of products and the performance of procedures Once a new product is developed and ready for use, there is often considerable education and training needed to safely introduce an instrument or procedure into clinical practice. The role of the physician and the PMA in education and training is critical, and direct physician involvement is needed in designing educational programs, without which a new tool may cause significant harm when introduced into general practice. Continued relationships between PMAs and industry are essential to the continued safe deployment of new medical devices and techniques to the practicing physician.

WHAT IS THE SUNSHINE LAW?

In addition to the different state laws, clinicians and drug and device manufacturers should be aware of a provision of the federal Patient Protection and Affordable Care Act (PPACA), which provides for transparency reports of industry payments to physicians to be publicly disclosed.[25] This provision, Section 6002 of the PPACA, is also known as the Physician Payment Sunshine Provision because it is based on the previously proposed, but never enacted, Physician Payment Sunshine Act. The PPACA requires that drug and medical device manufacturers report payments made to physicians to the Secretary of the Department of Health and Human Services but also requires the Secretary, in turn, to provide these required payment disclosure reports to the public through an Internet Web site that is searchable and in a format that is clear and understandable.

The PPACA defines "payment or other transfer of value broadly to mean "a transfer of anything of value." However, the following payments or transfers of value are exempt from disclosure:

- Payments or transfer of anything of value made indirectly to a physician through a third party, where the manufacturer is unaware of the identity of the physician
- Payments less than $10, unless the total amount paid to a physician during a calendar year exceeds $100
- Product samples that are not intended to be sold and are intended for patient use
- Educational materials that directly benefit patients or are intended for patient use
- The loan of a medical device for a short-term trial period that does not exceed 90 days
- Items or services provided under a contractual warranty, including the replacement of a medical device, where the terms of the warranty are set forth in the purchase or lease agreement for the medical device
- A transfer of anything of value to a physician when the physician is a patient and not acting in a professional capacity
- Discounts and rebates
- In-kind items used for charity
- A dividend or other profit distribution from ownership or investment interest in a publicly traded security or mutual fund.

Although the PPACA requires information to be made public, it treats payments to physicians assisting in the research and development of new drugs and devices differently. The Secretary does not publish payment information on the Web site until the FDA approves or clears the drug, device, biologic, or medical supply or[2] 4 years after the date of the payment to the doctor, whichever happens first.[1]

Drug and device manufacturers may face significant penalties for noncompliance with the reporting requirements, even if inadvertent. Under the PPACA, a manufacturer that fails to submit the required information in a timely manner "shall be subject to a civil money penalty of not less than $1,000, but not more than $10,000." If a manufacturer knowingly fails to submit the required information in a timely manner, the manufacturer "shall be subject to a civil money penalty of not less than $10,000, but not more than $100,000" for each payment not reported.

Many in the industry hoped that the federal PPACA would preempt the various state laws on this subject. However, the PPACA's preemption clause does not preempt any state statute or regulation that requires disclosure or reporting of information that is "not of the type required to be disclosed or reported" under the PPACA. It only preempts those state laws that are similar or weaker. As a result, drug and device manufacturers not only have to comply with the federal reporting and disclosure requirements imposed under the PPACA but also with the various and additional requirements of the States. There is a cost to industry for this collecting and reporting of information.

Drug and device manufacturers have time to prepare for the new federal disclosure requirements while also complying with the state laws. Under the PPACA, the Secretary is required to establish regulations and procedures for the submission of the payment information by October 1, 2011. Drug and device manufacturers must begin collecting and recording payment information on January 1, 2012 and the first disclosure of payments to physicians made during the preceding year must be submitted to the Secretary on or about March 31, 2013.

HOW SHOULD THE PIR EVOLVE?

The public expects access to new treatments. Its appetite for innovation has been bolstered by the constant attention given by the press to new treatments and by the promise from researchers of continuing advances.[26]

The objectives of companies in their relationships to academia often vary according to the size of the company. Large pharmaceutical companies see great value in access to academic talent, ideas, and research tools and deemphasize the importance of discrete inventions and patentable discoveries. In contrast, smaller companies, especially those that develop devices and diagnostic techniques, see greater value in obtaining late-stage technology (ie, products that are near clinical trial) and that are closer to market. These companies derive considerable value from their association with reputable institutions and investigators, which validates their efforts to raise venture capital and the potential value of the company and its product. Venture investors in these entities reinforce the importance of establishing the investigator's full commitment and making it public and visible. The most common vehicle used to assure such commitment is equity or stock options assigned to the investigator and, with increasing frequency, to the institution where the work is performed. Stock or options in young companies are affordable, because they become valuable only if the company and product become successful. Active participation by the investigator in the commercialization process is viewed as essential in creating value. This participation creates a powerful but controversial incentive for the investigator and has proved to be one of the most difficult issues for academic centers to manage.

AMCs vary in the stance they have taken toward relationships with industry. Many universities formally encourage entrepreneurial activity, but, informally, personal attitudes vary widely at these same institutions. This institutional posturing creates uncertainty within the academic community, complicates negotiations with companies, and inhibits effective transfer of technology. An open, informed, transparent, and timely process must be used to decide the terms of engagement and the protections that are required to prevent conflicts of interest, excessive secrecy, and other threats to academic independence.

Alternative forms of organizations will be required if the full potential of academic-industrial collaboration is to be realized, especially for research in basic biology and disease mechanisms. Such organizations are not new. Several universities have developed freestanding research institutes or foundations to house, manage, and isolate different kinds of research from the main activities of the institution. Examples are the Draper and Lincoln laboratories and the Whitehead Institute for Biomedical Research, all at the Massachusetts Institute of Technology; the Applied Physics Laboratory at the Johns Hopkins University; and the Wisconsin Alumni Research Foundation of the University of Wisconsin-Madison.[27] These freestanding entities have been able to control the 2-way flow of personnel and information (into and out of the parent university) without compromising the primary mission of either. Several novel public-private collaborations have been formed with the goal of accelerating the pace of basic discovery and its translation into practice. This model of organization grew out of the realization that neither industry nor academia could achieve what they desired without reaching out to others. Each set of relationships overcame critical questions of mutual respect and governance, and their structures allow the control of intellectual property, encouraging free inquiry and supporting the dissemination of new findings, and yet remain compatible with eventual commercialization.

Supporters of strict oversight of PIR believe that, for faculty members who wish to found a company or play an active part in one, these goals may best be obtained by taking part-time appointments or leaves of absence. A clear separation of academic roles from company roles is essential. AMCs must set a high standard for their faculty, even though such a policy may prove unpopular. In practice, this means that an individual faculty member should be required to choose between making a primary commitment to the company or to the AMC without the option of a commitment to both. This approach forces a choice between the relative security afforded by the AMC and the hope of rewards in the commercial world.

Supporters of PIR do not think that overly restrictive enforcement of the separation of physician and industry is beneficial. They note that industry funding can be separated from product bias and be firewall protected to:

1. Support CME as a means to improve quality of care and outcomes
2. Accelerate translation of science to the clinical care setting
3. Support needed scientific and clinical research, as well as career development of young scientists
4. Improve communication to patients about the benefits and risks of pharmaceutical/medical device products and equipment
5. Improve patient and physician adherence and compliance to pharmaceutical and device guidelines
6. Address gaps in patient communication and education.

The importance of a relationship between industry and clinicians was detailed in a recent editorial by Don K. Nakayama,[28] MD, MBA, Chairman of the Department of Surgery at Mercer University School of Medicine. He identified the misperceptions and myths that have led some AMCs and organizations to adopt such restrictive policies on industry interactions.[29] In his editorial, Dr Nakayama comes to the defense of industry-physician relationships by examining the economic, ethical, and legal foundations for conflict of interest restrictions between physicians and pharmaceutical and medical device industries.

One of the first problems with restrictive policies between physicians and industry that Dr Nakayama identified were that some of the regulations grew from alleged, and some from real, conflicts of interest involving both drug and device trials.

Dr Nakayama stated that "scientific misconduct, fraud, and dishonesty are noteworthy because of their rarity." Many policymakers overreacted by installing restrictive policies for events that are extremely rare. Policymakers did not consider the other consequences created by such policies, which are now chilling the collaboration between physicians and industry.

Dr Nakayama believes that, although some restrictions, such as payment disclosure, are reasonable, making "a total purge of any and all potential financial conflicts of interest is overkill." This approach is unnecessary. There needs to be more discussion about "an appropriate middle ground that acknowledges the rights of industry, physicians, residents, medical students, patients, and the public to the benefits that reasonable interactions between industry and clinicians may provide."

THE FUTURE

The future of working relationships between industry and clinicians remains uncertain. There have been examples of abuse of these relationships in the past. However, the value of relationships remains clear. Transparency is necessary so that everyone is aware of any potential financial conflicts. However, overly restrictive policies that eliminate those with industry relationships from university employment, specific patient care activities, or professional association leadership seem to be too restrictive and may impede the progress in medicine that has been so beneficial in the past.

REFERENCES

1. Nukols TK, Escarce JJ. Residency work-hour reform. A cost analysis including preventable adverse events. J Gen Intern Med 2005;20:873–8.
2. Campbell EG, Gruwn RL, Mountford J, et al. A national survey of physician-industry relationships. N Engl J Med 2007;356:1742–50.
3. Campbell EG, Rao SR, Desroches CM, et al. Physician professionalism and changes in physician-industry relationships from 2004–2009. Arch Intern Med 2010;170:1820–6.
4. National Physicians Alliance. Physicians should separate themselves from the pharmaceutical industry. Available at: http://npalliance.org/blog/2011/02/19/physicians-should-separate-themselves-from-the-pharmaceutical-industry. Accessed July 31, 2011.
5. Brennan TA, Rothman DJ, Blank L, et al. Health industry practices that create conflict of interest. JAMA 2006;295:429–33.
6. Barro J, Beaulieu N. Selection and improvement: physician responses to financial incentives. Working paper 10017. Available at: http://www.nber.org/papers/W100017. Accessed July 31, 2011.
7. Casebeer L, Bennett N, Kristofoco R, et al. Physician internet medical information seeking and on-line continuing education use patterns. J Contin Educ Health Prof 2002;22:33–42.
8. Mazamanian PE, Davis DA. Continuing medical education and the physician as a learner. Guide to evidence. JAMA 2002;288:1057–60.
9. Fordis M, King JE, Ballantyne CM, et al. Comparison of the instructional efficacy of internet-based CME with live interactive CME workshops. JAMA 2005;294:1043–51.
10. Groves KE, Sketris I, Teh SE. Prescription drug samples – does this marketing strategy counteract policies for quality use of medications. J Clin Pharm Ther 2003;28:259–71.

11. LaViolette PA. Medical devices and conflict of interest: unique issues and an industry code to address them. Cleve Clin J Med 2007;74(Suppl 2):526–8.
12. Inglehart JK. Finding money for health care reform – rooting out waste, fraud and abuse. N Engl J Med 2009;261:229–31.
13. Brody H, Light DW. Efforts to undermine public health. The inverse benefit law: how drug makers undermine patient safety and public health. Am J Public Health 2011;101:399–404.
14. Mitka M. New "law" attempts to exploit strategies drug makers use to sway prescribing. JAMA 2011;305:1083–4.
15. AAMC issues new guidelines to address conflict of interest in clinical care. Available at: https://www.aamc.org/newsroom/newsreleases/2010/136226/100630.html. Accessed July 31, 2011.
16. Washington University Physicians. Washington University School of Medicine in St Louis (MO). Conflict of interest on clinical care – policy on pharmaceutical and medical device industry relationships. Available at: http://wuphysicians.wustl.edu/page.aspx?pageID=251. Accessed July 31, 2011.
17. Rothman DJ, MacDonald WJ, Berkowitz CD, et al. Professional medical associations and their relationship with industry. A proposal for controlling conflict of interest. JAMA 2009;301:1367–72.
18. Policy and Medicine. Pooled CME funding may be a road to nowhere. Available at: http://www.policymed.com/2011/04/pooled-cme-funding-a-may-be-a-road-to-no-where.html. Accessed July 31, 2011.
19. Bodenheimer T, Fernandez A. High and rising health care costs, part 4: can costs be controlled while preserving quality. Ann Intern Med 2005;143:26–31.
20. The American College of Rheumatology. Medical professional society relationships with industry: a joint statement. Available at: www.rheumatology.org/about/pma.pdf. Accessed July 31, 2011.
21. Chatterji AK, Fabrizio KR, Mitchell W, et al. Physician-industry cooperation in the medical device industry. Health Aff 2008;27:1532–42.
22. Society of American Gastrointestinal and Endoscopic Surgeons. SAGES statement on relationships between professional medical associations and industry. Available at: http://www.sages.org/publication/id/COI/. Accessed July 31, 2011.
23. Steinbrook R. Controlling conflicts of interest – proposals from the Institute of Medicine. N Engl J Med 2009;360:2160–3.
24. Masia N. Archive. The cost of developing a new drug. Available at: http://www.America.gov http://www.america.gov/st/econ-english/2008/April/20080429230904myleen0.5233981.html. Accessed July 31, 2011.
25. Katz PO. The new health-care law and what it means for clinical gastroenterology. Am J Gastroenterol 2010;105:1460–5.
26. US Food and Drug Administration (FDA). Consumers (medical devices). Available at: http://www.fda.gov/MedicalDevices/ResourcesforYou/Consumers/default.htm. Accessed July 31, 2011.
27. Johns MM, Barnes M, Florencio PS. Restoring balance to industry-academia relationships in an era of institutional financial conflicts of interest. JAMA 2003;289:741–6.
28. Nakayama DK. In defense of industry-physician relationships. Am Surg 2010;76:987–94.
29. Baerlocher MO, Millward SF, Cardella JF. Conflicts of interest in the development of new international medical devices. J Interv Radiol 2009;20:309–13.

Demonstrating Value: Registries and Beyond

Samuel R. Walters, BS

KEYWORDS

• Registries • Quality • Gastroenterology • Reimbursement
• Safety • EHR

The Agency for Health Research and Quality (AHRQ) defines a patient registry as "an organized system that uses observational study methods to collect uniform data (clinical and other) to evaluate specified outcomes for a population defined by a particular disease, condition, or exposure, and that serves a predetermined scientific, clinical, or policy purpose(s)." Specific purposes of patient registries identified by AHRQ include measuring quality of care, studying the nature of disease, examining effectiveness of treatments, and monitoring safety.[1] Registries have additionally been used to support public policy,[2] create qualification channels for reimbursement,[3] and to identify potential clinical trial opportunities using observational data.[4] As the health care landscape has evolved, the purpose and scope of patient registries is expanding, creating opportunities for providers, payors, and patients to assess the value of health care services, compare the effectiveness of treatments that share an indication, test and validate outcome measures, and monitor patient safety.

Patient registries have continued to evolve to meet needs and challenges in health care. Medical societies and associations continue to assess the market, and develop and improve their registries to assist members in meeting new standards and expectations and to thrive in practice. By addressing federal health care legislation and evolving payor policies, providing a vehicle for comparative effectiveness research and product safety monitoring, and taking advantage of and supporting electronic health record adoption, patient registries will continue to exist as valuable resources in improving the quality and affordability of care.

MEETING FEDERAL REQUIREMENTS

The United States has the most expensive health care system in the world, with an average per capita expenditure of $7290, accounting for approximately 16% of gross domestic product (GDP) as of 2007.[5] The Congressional Budget Office has estimated that, without significant policy changes, health care expenditures will account for 25% of GDP in 2025, and 49% of GDP by 2082.[6] However, despite the nation's outsized

The author has nothing to disclose.
American Gastroenterological Association, 4930 Del Ray Avenue, Bethesda, MD 20814, USA
E-mail address: swalters@gastro.org

Gastrointest Endoscopy Clin N Am 22 (2012) 135–145
doi:10.1016/j.giec.2011.08.010   **giendo.theclinics.com**

health care spending compared with other post-industrial nations, it has been ranked last in nearly all quality indicators in numerous studies.[5,7,8]

In an attempt to restrain health care expenditure growth and improve access and quality of care, on March 23, 2010, President Obama signed the Patient Protection and Affordable Care Act into law. Key components of this legislation include improving access to coverage through the creation of state-based health exchanges; a requirement for all US citizens to have health care coverage; a requirement for all employers with more than 50 full-time employees to offer health care coverage; and the creation of premium and cost-sharing subsidies for individual beneficiaries and employers. In addition, the act includes numerous provisions relating to the administration of the Medicare program, including a restructuring of Medicare Advantage payments, an Independent Payment Advisory Board responsible for creating proposals to reduce per capita Medicare expenditures, support for the creation of accountable care organizations (ACOs), and support for comparative effectiveness research through the establishment of the Patient-Centered Outcomes Research Institute.[9] These provisions, as well as the others present in the act, have the potential to radically restructure how health care is delivered, measured, and reimbursed in the United States, with many provisions already taking effect and affecting policy and practice.

The Center for Medicare and Medicaid Services (CMS) has planned and executed numerous demonstration projects and policy changes to support the movement to value-based health care, a model in which health care quality and costs are factored to determine the overall value of services delivered. Through projects to evaluate new care delivery models, such as the evaluation of the Patient-Centered Medical Home model, pay-for-reporting and pay-for-performance reimbursement policies including the CMS Physician Quality Reporting System (PQRS), and tools for public transparency and comparison such as the Compare websites for hospital, nursing home, and physician performance, the CMS is exploring new ways to provide patients with high-quality health care that is delivered for the most competitive costs.[10] These emerging models represent both significant opportunities and threats to health care providers and organizations, given their capacity to reshape health care delivery and reimbursement.

Patient registries can serve as valuable tools in meeting these challenges and demonstrating an accurate representation of quality and efficiency. An example of this is the creation of the registry reporting option for PQRS program. This quality measure reporting system was established through a provision of the 2006 Tax Relief and Health Care Act, and has continued each year since. PQRS requires providers to satisfactorily report a minimum number of quality measures to receive an incentive payment for participation. In addition, the Medicare Improvement for Patients and Providers Act mandates that the names of providers who successfully submit to the PQRS be provided on the CMS Web site.[11] In 2009, a total of $234 million in incentives were paid to 119,804 providers in 12,647 practices.[12]

PQRS reporting was initially only available through the reporting of quality codes on Medicare claims. However, in 2008, the option to report PQRS measures through a qualifying patient registry became available. Registries meeting CMS qualification process standards are approved to submit quality measure data on behalf of providers, and are additionally required to provide feedback quality reports to participants.[13] Since the introduction of the registry reporting mechanism, reporting rates have increased, and providers submitting to PQRS using the registry option were more likely to earn an incentive payment, and earn a higher incentive payment, than providers submitting using other options such as claims submission.[12]

In 2010, the American Gastroenterological Association (AGA) Digestive Health Outcomes Registry (AGA Registry), a national digestive disease patient registry, achieved CMS approval as a PQRS-qualified registry for reporting 2009 measures. Seeking to provide a simple solution to meeting PQRS requirements, the registry incorporated the PQRS hepatitis C measures group, a collection of 8 measures of quality in hepatitis C treatment. The measures group reporting option through PQRS in 2009 required that a provider report all measures in the group for a minimum of 30 patients, of which 2 must be Medicare Fee for Service, or report the group for at least 80% of the provider's Medicare Fee for Service population. By becoming a qualified registry, the AGA Registry was able to successfully report quality measures on behalf of 46 providers, qualifying them for a potential 2% reimbursement bonus for all 2009 Medicare Fee for Service claims. The registry continues to offer this option for 2010 reporting, because it offers providers a way to meet their quality reporting needs in a minimally burdensome manner, and additionally serves as a driver for registry participation.[14] Programs such as PQRS will continue to serve as important mechanisms by which health care providers can demonstrate a commitment to quality through guideline-driven practice and efficient use of resources. As the federal government continues to seek ways to control rising health care expenditures, patient registries will serve as a vital channel through which detailed clinical data and nationally endorsed measures can drive policy and support providers as they seek reimbursement incentives and avoid penalties.

Additional opportunities for meeting federal requirements through patient registries exist in the standards established by CMS for ACOs. Medicare ACO standards include the creation of the Medicare Shared Savings Program, which is designed to improve care coordination and communications between providers. CMS has identified 65 process and outcome measures that will be used to assess the quality of patient care within the ACO setting, and has proposed that, in addition to claims-based submission of these measures, data collection will also be approved using a tool designed for clinical quality measure reporting, which includes quality-focused patient registries. In addition, measure #23 in the ACO measure set is a measure of patient registry use in the ACO. Using patient registries as data collection, measurement, and reporting systems can assist providers in meeting the ACO standards and participating in the Shared Savings Program.[15]

Patient registries are well positioned to support coverage with evidence development (CED) studies, as outlined in a national coverage determination in 2006. CED studies collect data to determine the appropriateness of treatments and improve the evidence base for expansion of payor coverage.[16] The American College of Cardiology's ICD (implantable cardioverter-defibrillator) Registry is an example of a patient registry used for CED studies on behalf of CMS. Established in 2006, the ICD Registry collects information about implantable cardioverting defibrillators, including physician training and inpatient outcomes. The registry was initially proposed because of the determination of CMS that "the available evidence does not provide a high degree of guidance to providers to target these devices to patients who will clearly derive benefit." Although randomized controlled trials showed clear benefit in ICDs as a primary prevention for sudden cardiac death, the differences in the median age of the Medicare population (70–75 years) and the trial populations were significant enough to warrant reconsideration of the evidence.

To address these questions, CMS proposed a national ICD registry in 2004, participation in which would be a condition for reimbursement for institutions performing implantations. After a workgroup was convened by the Heart Rhythm Society to determine registry design, the National Cardiovascular Data Registry (NCDR) was selected as the administrator of, and data repository for, the registry. Because participation in the registry was mandated for reimbursement, nearly 100% of eligible sites were enrolled within 4 months, and more than 400,000 procedures have been documented.[1]

Data from the registry were used to show that 22.5% of implants between 2006 and 2009 did not meet the American Heart Association, American College of Cardiology, European Society of Cardiology, and Heart Rhythm Society guidelines for appropriateness.[17] The study further showed that disparities in physician training could be a probable factor in non–evidence-based implantations.[18] The ICD Registry has since been updated to include lead data (including lead failures), pediatric ICD implantations, and additional quality measures beyond the registry's original scope,[19] and continues to be used to determine whether ICD implantations are indicated for Medicare beneficiaries.[20]

Quality, efficiency, and appropriateness continue to drive federal decisions regarding coverage and reimbursement, as well as recognition of emerging care environments including ACOs and patient-centered medical homes, and registries have the potential to continue their unique role in supporting providers in this evolving landscape. Many federal health reform efforts have proactively included registry options and consideration, which is a positive sign that they will remain a viable quality measurement and reporting source as health care continues to be shaped by legislation.

PRIVATE PAYOR COLLABORATION

Private health care payors have embraced several of the trends set by the federal government, seeking to lower health care costs per beneficiary while determining which of their providers are delivering outcomes that meet performance thresholds. Programs such as United Healthcare's UnitedHealth Premium program use quality measures derived from health care claims data to assess individual provider quality of care and cost efficiency, and provide benefits such as premium directory listings.[21] Patient registries capturing the necessary quality measures for these programs can provide clinicians with the capability to meet the requirements of multiple health payor programs, rather than devote effort separately and incur unnecessary redundant resource consumption.

In another example, Aetna's Institutes of Excellence and Institutes of Quality programs offer a designation for facilities and providers that demonstrate an ability to provide high-quality, cost-effective care. Additional requirements include that care is delivered in an accredited facility with appropriate infrastructure including an in-house data-driven quality improvement program, and reporting of the Leapfrog Hospital Survey or an equivalent patient safety and quality reporting program.[22] Although such programs are currently offered as incentives, these programs will become the standard by which providers are measured in the coming decade, and, subsequently, by which reimbursement is determined.

The Aetna Institutes of Quality Cardiac Care Facilities program is an example of a health payor program that integrates with patient registries to measure quality of care. Facilities applying for recognition through this program are required to participate in, and report from, the American College of Cardiology's NCDR, and the Society of Thoracic Surgeons (STS) National Database. Established in 1997, the NCDR is a national quality measurement registry with more than 2200 participating hospitals and encompassing a suite of 6 cardiovascular registries: CathPCI Registry, which measures quality in cardiac stenting procedures; CARE Registry, capturing carotid stenting and endarterectomy procedures; ACTION Registry, for acute coronary syndrome; ICD Registry, covering patients receiving implantable cardioverting defibrillators; IMPACT Registry, which includes adults and pediatrics with congenital heart conditions; and the PINNACLE Network, a registry measuring outpatient quality in cardiovascular care.[23] The STS National Database was established in 1989 and supports quality improvement in thoracic surgery, with 3 components: adult cardiac, general thoracic, and congenital heart surgery.[24] Applicants for the Aetna program must successfully report all measures supported by the NCDR, as well as their STS STAR rating (Quality Aggregate Rating) score.[25] By using these registries to measure, monitor, and report quality, Aetna providers are able to meet requirements to become recognized for their commitment to improving outcomes in a cost-effective manner.

Given the quality measurement goals of patient registries, there is significant opportunity for integration with other payment incentive programs. The Bridges to Excellence (BTE) program through the Health Care Incentives Improvement Institute (HCI3) provides recognition programs that can lead to per patient incentive payments from participating health plans. The programs include recognition for conditions including asthma, cardiac care, depression, diabetes, hypertension, coronary artery disease, spine care, and chronic obstructive pulmonary disease.[26] The National Committee for Quality Assurance (NCQA) provides quality measurement programs for recognition in the treatment of back pain, diabetes, and heart/stroke.[27] These programs rely on clinical data to measure quality in the respective clinical domains, and compute aggregate quality scores to determine recognition status. Patient registries that already capture these data could be effectively integrated to allow registry participants to meet recognition needs across multiple recognition programs, and thereby see potential gains in reimbursement across health payors.

As existing sources of guidelines-driven quality measurement, patient registries have the capacity to meet reporting requirements for such programs using clinically derived, detailed data based on endorsed and validated measures, rather than via claims data that do not provide an accurate picture of patient care. In addition, registries can serve as a single source for capturing and reporting health payor program quality data, reducing redundancy and providing consistency of measurement across payors and care environments. Registries including the American Society for Clinical Oncology's Quality Oncology Practice Initiative (QOPI) have already formed partnerships with 13 health payors to provide benefits to participating facilities who meet quality thresholds in oncologic care.[28] The AGA is also currently working with numerous health payors and quality measurement and reporting organizations to design incentive programs that are driven by quality measures reported by the AGA Registry, including inflammatory bowel disease (IBD) management and colorectal cancer prevention (CRC-P) outcome measures.[29] As health plans move toward the formation of tiered and narrow networks, pay for quality programs, and further recognition and designation programs, and the use of clinical data provided by registries to provide fair and accurate quality reporting will continue to grow.

COMPARATIVE EFFECTIVENESS RESEARCH

Comparative effectiveness research compares two or more methods, products, or services, and examines their relative efficacy in the treatment of disease. Traditional research typically focuses on only one treatment options. The ARRA (American Recovery and Reinvestment Act) has allocated $1.1 billion to fund comparative effectiveness research at the AHRQ and the National Institutes of Health (NIH).[30] In addition, the Patient Protection and Affordable Care Act (PPACA) of 2010 established the Patient-Centered Outcomes Research Institute (PCORI), an independent nonprofit organization tasked with identifying research to give patients a more accurate picture of their treatment options, preventive care, and the science underlying them. As part of this mission, PCORI will commission research that compares the relative efficacy of treatments and provide this information to health consumers and providers.[31]

Following ARRA's execution, the Institute of Medicine (IOM) identified 100 priority areas in comparative effectiveness research. Of special note are the gastrointestinal and hepatological topics included as priorities:

- Comparative effectiveness of upper endoscopy utilization and frequency for patients with gastroesophageal reflux disease on morbidity, quality of life, and diagnosis of esophageal carcinoma
- Compare the effectiveness of different strategies for introducing biologics into the treatment algorithm for inflammatory disease, including Crohn disease, ulcerative colitis, rheumatoid arthritis, and psoriatic arthritis
- Compare the effectiveness of alternative clinical management strategies for hepatitis C, including alternative duration of therapy for patients based on viral genomic profile and patient risk factors (eg, behavior-related risk factors)
- Compare the effectiveness of new screening technologies (such as fecal immunochemical tests and computed tomography [CT] colonography) and usual care (fecal occult blood tests and colonoscopy) in preventing colorectal cancer
- Compare the effectiveness of genetic and biomarker testing and usual care in preventing and treating breast, colorectal, prostate, lung, and ovarian cancer, and possibly other clinical conditions for which promising biomarkers exist.

There is significant opportunity for patient registries to support comparative effectiveness using observational datasets. Randomized clinical trials are the gold standard for evidence development, but lack the ability to capture prospective data from all care environments and to monitor the ongoing evolution of treatment and disease. Registries can provide an alternative data collection and measurement mechanism that builds the data necessary to inform decision making in a rapid fashion and drive comparative effectiveness research. The outcomes of these studies have the capacity to inform physicians and policy makers of the optimal care choices available for patients, and to increase cost-effectiveness in the system.

PRODUCT SAFETY MONITORING

Quality measurement registries can serve as a mechanism for observational monitoring of product safety events in the postmarket phase of the medical product lifecycle. Although such registries may not be explicitly designed for this purpose, their capture of product information for quality measurement can often be repurposed to provide information about product performance through observational study. Such study provides opportunities for safety monitoring and evaluation not present within traditional clinical trials, including comparative product performance and safety within populations sometimes excluded from trials, including women, children, and the elderly. These registries can also monitor and report the safety of products in patients who are treated with polypharmacy regimens, another population frequently excluded from clinical trials. By planning for product safety monitoring in the process of registry development, mechanisms for signal detection methodologies can be incorporated and used to detect adverse events and unanticipated outcomes prospectively, providing an ongoing mechanism for measurement across large and diverse populations not captured through trials.[1]

The NCDR's CathPCI Registry, although originally designed for quality and outcomes measurement, was used as the data source for a study to assess the comparative safety of hemostasis devices following cardiac catheterization, in response to reports to the US Food and Drug Administration (FDA) of vascular complications and injury attributed to these devices. Using procedure data from 59 institutions and comprising 13,878 catheterizations, individual assessment was conducted of 2 collagen plug hemostasis devices: Angio-Seal and VasoSeal. Two other devices were assessed: Chito-Seal and the Syvek NT Patch, both approved by the FDA for wound dressing, but not for hemostasis. The results of this study indicated that there were significantly higher adverse events associated with VasoSeal use compared with Angio-Seal.[32] As a result of this study, the VasoSeal device was subsequently removed from the market. The NCDR has continued to collaborate with the FDA to design further studies, including monitoring ICD and atrial fibrillation ablation safety.[33] Safety monitoring opportunities in gastroenterology could similarly be enabled through the use of prospective quality registries, allowing for assessment of the safety of pharmaceutical regimens, procedures, and devices.

INTEGRATION WITH ELECTRONIC HEALTH RECORDS

An additional factor affecting the delivery of health care and availability of information is electronic health record (EHR) adoption. The ARRA in 2009 set in place a mandate for CMS to create an incentive program that provides additional reimbursement to providers who adopt and show that they are meaningfully using EHRs. The criterion for meaningful use of an EHR includes showing the ability to exchange information to improve quality of care, such as through care coordination, and the capability of quality measure reporting.[34] These requirements contributed to a steady climb in the number of providers and facilities using EHRs, and this trend is expected to continue for the duration of the incentive program.[35] This increase in connectivity requires broader development and adoption of standards to increase health data exchange and interpretation than are presently available. Although standards for health information exist, there are deficits in common clinical terminology, system interface standards, and minimum data sets. Efforts to bridge these gaps have increased considerably since the adoption of the ARRA, and are expected to continue in the coming years.[36]

The Guideline Advantage™ program, a joint program of the American Cancer Society, American Diabetes Association, American Heart Association, and American Stroke association, incorporates guidelines and measurements specific to these specialties directly into EHRs. Through customized measurement tools and ongoing assessment of measures, the program enables clinicians to document and measure care in real time, and assess guideline compliance. In addition, the program allows clinicians to capture the core clinical quality measures necessary to meet the clinical quality measurement requirements for meaningful use.[37] Guideline Advantage has integrated Forward Health Group, GEMMS, and New Century Health's EHRs as of August 2011, and also provides a mechanism by which practices with other EHRs can add registry functionality to their systems.[38]

In gastroenterology, the AGA Registry has been successfully incorporated into gMed's gCare version 4.0. Registry participants using gMed can now directly collect and submit data from their gCare EHR, with no required customization. The integration of the registry within a gastroenterology-specific system provides a standardized approach to the capture, review, and measurement of clinical results, and provides gastroenterologists with guidelines-driven quality measurement directly at the point of care.[39] The AGA Registry has additionally partnered with FIGMD, Inc., a clinical systems integrator, to provide custom integration for EHRs that do not have the registry directly incorporated. Using this approach, practices work with FIGMD to identify the data resident in their EHRs that are necessary to calculate the quality and outcome measures supported by the registry. FIGMD identifies any gaps in documentation, and assists the practice in updating their templates and databases to include the necessary data. Once integrated, the practice automatically submits data to the registry with no intervention required on the part of practice staff.[40] The inclusion of data necessary to capture these measures has an inherent effect of modifying practice workflow to ensure that patients are cared for in accordance with the guidelines on which these measures are based.

The integration of patient registries into EHRs and other clinical systems represents an opportunity to influence the degree of support they provide specific to gastroenterology, by capturing the data necessary to calculate quality and outcome measures based on clinical guidelines. Their inclusion within a clinical system requires that the information required for calculating measures be incorporated into the system, providing clinicians with the ability to document and assess guidelines-driven care. In addition, the inclusion of these data and measures enables the creation of custom templates, and the inclusion of specialty-designed care pathways, providing further tools to improve documentation, measurement, and management of patient care that are sensitive to the needs of a given specialty.

SUMMARY

Although quality measurement registries have traditionally been designed and operated with the primary goal of supporting performance, quality, and outcomes measurement and improvement in practice, they are increasingly being expanded and repurposed to address emerging and persistent issues in health care delivery. Following the examples set by other medical specialties, gastroenterology is positioned to use registries to adapt to the changing health care environment and provide optimal care for patients. The inclusion of quality and outcome measures important to both the specialty and to payors, purchasers, and patients will provide gastroenterologists with a mechanism to demonstrate value, deliver guidelines-driven care, and meet the challenges of reimbursement structures including pay-for-performance, narrow networks, and tiered networks, and novel care delivery structures such as patient-centered medical homes and ACOs. Meeting these requirements and adapting to this landscape is the only way to ensure the ongoing viability of gastroenterological practice and create a realistic care delivery and coordination system for the specialty.

Concurrent with the restructuring of payment and care delivery is the increasing adoption of EHRs and interconnectivity of clinical systems. To provide tangible benefit to gastroenterologists and enable the delivery of optimal patient care, these systems must store, communicate, and provide actionable decision support that is driven by approved clinical guidelines, and informed by the ongoing measurement of adherence and outcomes. Challenges remain in the integration of ancillary clinical systems such as endoscopic reporting systems, and the identification and addition of crucial data elements to measure and deliver evidence-based care will inform the standards necessary for interconnectivity. When the data necessary for measurement and improvement are fully integrated and exchanged between systems, opportunities for the development of care pathways and decision support systems will be greatly enhanced, providing further mechanisms for delivering optimal patient care.

Patient registries additionally offer the opportunity to support product safety and comparative effectiveness research, which are topics of increasing interest and for which there have been limited mechanisms for assessing in the US environment. Through prospective data capture and signal monitoring, registries will continue to serve as crucial tools in the detection and evaluation of product safety events and adverse outcomes, as already demonstrated among several specialties. Within gastroenterology, there exists opportunity for the ongoing assessment of pharmacotherapy regimens, including complex cases in which polytherapy is used or underrepresented populations are treated. Further, capturing performance and outcomes across procedure, device, and drug types will allow opportunities for supporting comparative effectiveness research, and provide gastroenterologists and patients with the necessary findings to determine optimal treatments, accurately assess potential risks, and demonstrate the value of treatment to payors.

Quality registries in gastroenterology are largely in their infancy, and it is likely that further uses for these programs will emerge in the coming years. By taking advantage of the existing opportunities identified by other specialties, and continuing to adopt registries to meet new challenges as they arise, registries will serve as important tools in supporting the practice and science of gastroenterology, informing policy makers, and, most importantly, helping to deliver the best care for patients.

REFERENCES

1. (Prepared by outcome DEcIDE Center [Outcome Sciences, Inc. dba Outcome] under Contract No. HHSA29020050035ITO1.) AHRQ Publication No. 07-EH001-1. In: Gliklich RE, Dreyer NA, editors. Registries for evaluating patient outcomes: a user's guide. Rockville (MD): Agency for Healthcare Research and Quality; 2007. p. 1–11, 79–85, 222–3.
2. Haynes T. It takes a community to grow good data. Children's Hospitals Today 2008.
3. The National Oncology PET Registry (NOPR). Available at: http://www.cancer petregistry.org/what.htm. Accessed July 24, 2011.
4. The National Lymphatic Disease and Lymphedema Registry. Available at: http://lymphaticresearch.org/main.php?menu=research&content=patient-reg-new. Accessed July 24, 2011.
5. Davis K, Schoen C, Stremikis K. Mirror, mirror on the wall: how the performance of the U.S. Health Care System compares internationally. The Commonwealth Fund; 2010. p. 1–10.
6. Orszag PR. CBO testimony: growth in healthcare costs, before the Committee on the Budget, United States Senate. The Congressional Budget Office; 2008.
7. Guyatt GH, Devereaux PJ, Lexchin J, et al. A systematic review of studies comparing health outcomes in Canada and the United States. Open Med 2007;1(1):e27–36.
8. Nolte E, McKee M. Measuring the health of nations: analysis of mortality amenable to health care. BMJ 2003;327(7424):1129.
9. Summary of new health reform law. Focus on Health Reform. The Henry J. Kaiser Family Foundation; 2011.
10. Roadmap for implementing value driven healthcare in the traditional Medicare fee-for-service program. Centers for Medicare and Medicaid Services, U.S. Department of Health and Human Services.
11. Overview: physician quality reporting system. Available at: https://www.cms.gov/PQRS/. Last updated April 20, 2011. Accessed July 23, 2011.
12. 2009 Reporting experience: Physician Quality Reporting System and electronic prescribing (eRx) incentive program. Centers for Medicare and Medicaid Studies; 2011. p. vi–vii, xv–xvi.

13. Alternative reporting mechanisms. Available at: https://www.cms.gov/PQRS/20_ AlternativeReportingMechanisms.asp#TopOfPage. Last updated May 31, 2011. Accessed July 23, 2011.
14. MedAssurant supports the American Gastroenterological Association's successful submission of 2010 PQRS quality measure data. Available at: http://med assurant.com/public-relations-article.aspx?id=60. Last updated March 17, 2011. Last accessed July 23, 2011.
15. Improving quality of care for Medicare patients: accountable care organizations. Available at: https://www.cms.gov/MLNProducts/downloads/ACO_Quality_Fact sheet_ICN906104.pdf. Accessed July 25, 2011.
16. National coverage determinations with data collection as a condition of coverage: coverage with evidence development. Available at: https://www.cms.gov/medicare-coverage-database/details/medicare-coverage-document-details.aspx?MCDId= 8&McdName=National+Coverage+Determinations+with+Data+Collection+as+ a+Condition+of+Coverage%3a+Coverage+with+Evidence+Development&mcd typename=Guidance+Documents&MCDIndexType=1&bc=BAAIAAAAAAAA&. Last updated July 12, 2006. Accessed July 25, 2011.
17. Al-Khatib SM, Hellkamp A, Curtis J, et al. Non-evidence-based ICD implantations in the United States. JAMA 2011;305(1):43–9.
18. Miller R. Nearly a quarter of ICD implants are not recommended by professional guidelines. Available at: http://www.theheart.org/article/1168527.do. Last updated January 4, 2011. Accessed July 25, 2011.
19. ICD Registry. Available at: https://www.ncdr.com/webncdr/ICD/Default_ssl.aspx. Accessed July 25, 2011.
20. About ICD Registry. Available at: http://www.ncdr.com/WebNCDR/ICD/ABOUT ICD.ASPX. Accessed July 25, 2011.
21. United Health Premium. Available at: https://www.unitedhealthcareonline.com/b2c/ CmaAction.do?channelId=a7b0465138a17210VgnVCM1000002f10b10a. Accessed July 25, 2011.
22. Aetna Institutes. Available at: http://www.aetna.com/healthcare-professionals/ quality-measurement/institutes.html. Accessed July 25, 2011.
23. About NCDR. Available at: http://www.ncdr.com/WebNCDR/COMMON/ABOUT US.ASPX. Accessed July 23, 2011.
24. STS National Database. Available at: http://sts.org/national-database. Accessed July 23, 2011.
25. Aetna Institutes of Quality Cardiac Care Facilities: program requirements. Available at: http://www.aetna.com/provider/data/AIOQCardiac_care_facility_program_ criteria.pdf. Accessed July 23, 2011.
26. Recognition programs. Available at: http://www.prometheuspayment.org/ recognition_programs. Accessed July 25, 2011.
27. Recognition. Available at: http://www.ncqa.org/tabid/74/Default.aspx. Accessed July 25, 2011.
28. QOPI Health Plan integration. Available at: http://qopi.asco.org/Health_Plan_ Program. Accessed July 25, 2011.
29. Partnering with health plans. Available at: http://www.gastro.org/practice/digestive-health-outcomes-registry/participating-in-the-aga-registry/health-plans. Accessed July 25, 2011.
30. Explaining health reform: what is comparative effectiveness research? Focus on health reform. The Henry J. Kaiser Family Foundation; 2009.
31. About PCORI. Available at: http://www.pcori.org/aboutus.html. Accessed July 25, 2011.

32. J Invasive Cardiol 2005;17(12):644–50.
33. IOM (Institute of Medicine). Public health effectiveness of the FDA 510(k) clearance process: measuring postmarket performance and other select topics: workshop report. Washington, DC: The National Academies Press; 2011. p. 25.
34. American Recovery and Reinvestment Act of 2009, 4 USC §4101 (2009).
35. Hsiao CJ, Hing E, Socey TC, et al. Electronic medical record/health record systems of office-based Physicians: United States, 2009 and preliminary 2010 state estimates. National Center for Health Statistics; 2010.
36. Bell KM. EHR incentive programs: interoperability 101. Available at: http://www.ehrincentive.com/2011/04/interoperability-101.html. Accessed July 25, 2011.
37. Frequently asked questions. Available at: http://www.guidelineadvantage.org/TGA/FAQ/FAQ_UCM_428664_FAQ.jsp. Accessed July 25, 2011.
38. Compatible vendors. Available at: http://www.guidelineadvantage.org/TGA/HowToParticipate/ParticipatingVendors/Compatible-Vendors_UCM_428647_Article.jsp. Accessed July 25, 2011.
39. gMed users can now submit data directly to the AGA Registry. Available at: http://gmed.com/newsfeed.asp?feed=gMedSubmitAGAreg. Accessed August 19, 2011.
40. AGA Now offers direct data submission from electronic medical records into registry. Available at: http://www.gastro.org/news/articles/2011/07/29/aga-now-offers-direct-data-submission-from-electronic-medical-records-into-registry. Updated July 29, 2011. Accessed August 19, 2011.

Index

Gastrointest Endoscopy Clin N Am 22 (2012) 147–154
doi:10.1016/S1052-5157(11)00133-4   **giendo.theclinics.com**
1052-5157/12/$ – see front matter © 2012 Elsevier Inc. All rights reserved.

Moving?

Make sure your subscription moves with you!

To notify us of your new address, find your **Clinics Account Number** (located on your mailing label above your name), and contact customer service at:

Email: journalscustomerservice-usa@elsevier.com

800-654-2452 (subscribers in the U.S. & Canada)
314-447-8871 (subscribers outside of the U.S. & Canada)

Fax number: 314-447-8029

Elsevier Health Sciences Division
Subscription Customer Service
3251 Riverport Lane
Maryland Heights, MO 63043

*To ensure uninterrupted delivery of your subscription, please notify us at least 4 weeks in advance of move.

Printed and bound by CPI Group (UK) Ltd, Croydon, CR0 4YY

03/10/2024

01040456-0014